EMERGENCY IMAGING

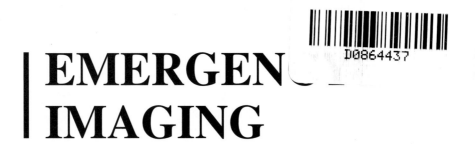

EMERGENCY IMAGING

R. Brooke Jeffrey, Jr., M.D.
Professor of Radiology
Chief of Abdominal Imaging
Stanford University School of Medicine
Stanford, California

Philip W. Ralls, M.D.
Professor of Radiology
University of Southern California School of Medicine, and
Los Angeles County and
University of Southern California
Medical Center
Los Angeles, California

Ann N. Leung, M.D.
Assistant Professor
Department of Radiology
Stanford University School of Medicine, and
Chief of Thoracic Imaging
Stanford University Medical Center
Stanford, California

Michael Brant-Zawadzki, M.D., F.A.C.R.
Medical Director
Department of Radiology
Director of MRI
Hoag Memorial Hospital Presbyterian, and
Clinical Professor of Diagnostic Radiology
Stanford University
Stanford, California

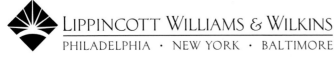
LIPPINCOTT WILLIAMS & WILKINS
PHILADELPHIA · NEW YORK · BALTIMORE

Acquisitions Editor: James D. Ryan
Developmental Editor: Brian Brown
Manufacturing Manager: Tim Reynolds
Production Manager: Liane Carita
Production Editor: Robin E. Cook
Cover Designer: Christine Jenny
Indexer: Ron Prottsman
Compositor: Maryland Composition
Printer: Maple Press

Printed in the United States of America

9 8 7 6 5 4 3 2 1

Library of Congress Cataloging-in-Publication Data

Emergency imaging / R. Brooke Jeffrey . . . [et al.].
    p.   cm.
    Includes bibliographical references and index.
    ISBN 0-7817-1592-X
    1, Diagnostic imaging.   2. Medical emergencies.   3. Emergency medicine.   I. Jeffrey, R. Brooke.
    [DNLM: 1. Diagnostic Imaging.   2. Emergencies.   3. Acute Disease. WN 180 E53   1999]
    RC78.7.D53E44   1999
    616.07′54—dc21
    DNLM/DLC
    for Library of Congress   98-31217
                                                                          CIP

Care has been taken to confirm the accuracy of the information presented and to describe generally accepted practices. However, the authors, editors, and publisher are not responsible for errors or omissions or for any consequences from application of the information in this book and make no warranty, expressed or implied, with respect to the contents of the publication.

The authors, editors, and publisher have exerted every effort to ensure that drug selection and dosage set forth in this text are in accordance with current recommendations and practice at the time of publication. However, in view of ongoing research, changes in government regulations, and the constant flow of information relating to drug therapy and drug reactions, the reader is urged to check the package insert for each drug for any change in indications and dosage and for added warnings and precautions. This is particularly important when the recommended agent is a new or infrequently employed drug.

Some drugs and medical devices presented in this publication have Food and Drug Administration (FDA) clearance for limited use in restricted research settings. It is the responsibility of the health care provider to ascertain the FDA status of each drug or device planned for use in their clinical practice.

To Stefanie, Catherine, Luke, and Elizabeth

Contents

Preface

Cross-sectional imaging with computed tomography (CT), ultrasound (US), and magnetic resonance imaging (MRI) plays a pivotal role in the evaluation of acutely ill and traumatized patients. There is an increasing awareness that early diagnosis in these patients with rapid triage to either medical or surgical therapy is critical to the delivery of cost-effective health care. Accurate diagnosis on the "front end" often results in reduced length of patient hospitalization and saves considerable cost by avoiding delays in instituting therapy and eliminating unnecessary surgery.

Cross-sectional imaging has recently undergone dramatic technological changes. During the past five years, newer pulse sequences, faster gradients, and contrast agents have had a significant impact on MRI. CT has undergone a major technological revolution with the advent of helical (spiral) CT. Color and power Doppler US are now routine in clinical practice. Due to the rapid pace of development in these modalities over the past few years, we felt that a concise reference guide highlighting newer protocols and state-of the art imaging would be useful both for residents on call and practicing radiologists. These technological advances, while improving imaging in any instances, lead to greater complexity in terms of scanning protocols. More imaging options now exist to evaluate acutely ill patients. Given this complexity, it is vitally important to make the correct choice of imaging modality and scanning parameters.

This book provides a concise overview of important clinical and imaging findings in patients undergoing emergency imaging. We have tried to focus on the most common and the most challenging problems in clinical practice. Our other main objectives are to concisely discuss optimal cross-sectional imaging techniques, to avoid technical errors, and to interpret pitfalls. The organization of the book parallels patient symptoms rather than using an organ system approach. It is our view that this structure more closely corresponds to the actual experience of practicing radiologists in the day-to-day clinical setting. Our aim is to provide practical imaging solutions to everyday clinical problems in acutely ill patients.

Acknowledgments

To Derick Yih for outstanding administrative and editorial assistance.

RBJ

To Betty Hemphill for superb research and administrative support.

PWR

I would like to thank Patricia Detton for her administrative assistance.

ANL

The gracious and efficient assistance of Robin Francis in the preparation of the neuroradiology chapters and figures in this book is greatly appreciated.

MBZ

1

Head Trauma

Michael Brant-Zawadzki

I. CLINICAL OVERVIEW

Head trauma remains one of the most common indications for cranial imaging, particularly in the urban emergency department setting. Before the development of cross-sectional imaging methodologies, plain x-rays and clinical findings alone were used for rapid diagnosis and urgent therapeutic interventions. Conventional angiography was used when extraaxial or intraaxial hematoma was suspected. The introduction of computed tomography (CT) had a major impact on the evaluation of victims of head trauma. In these days of cost–benefit concerns, one of the earliest demonstrations of a positive impact on cost–benefit analysis was the use of CT for detecting subdural hematomas and other intracranial injury. CT has virtually eliminated the use of skull x-rays and emergency angiograms in patients with head trauma. Magnetic resonance imaging (MRI) has expanded the imaging approach for evaluating head trauma, particularly in the subacute time frame. Detection of shear injury or subtle extraaxial collections, evaluation of intracranial vessel injury (post-traumatic pseudoaneurysm or cavernous-carotid fistula), and even the detection of subtle basal brain contusions not seen initially on CT have all been made easier by MRI.

II. IMAGING STRATEGY

Computed tomography has become the first step in evaluating patients with acute head injury. The urge to start with plain x-rays (seen especially with the emergency medicine physi-cian) particularly in cases of "minor" head trauma should be resisted. Negative plain x-rays may lead to a false sense of security. Indeed, any patient with head trauma in whom x-rays are considered for "medical-legal reasons," warrants a CT study (Figs. 1 and 2). In the past, multidisciplinary groups developed indications for obtaining plain x-rays following head trauma, which have subsequently been transposed to the CT examination. These indications include focal neurologic findings, altered level of consciousness after trauma, palpable depressed skull fracture, clinical signs of basilar fracture ("raccoon" eyes, blood behind the ear drums), evidence of cerebrospinal fluid (CSF) leak from the nose or ear, and penetrating head injury. Additionally, significant facial fracture (an entity not included in this review) can often be associated with intracranial injury—particularly when complex LeForte or tripod injuries occur (Fig. 3). Therefore, such facial trauma when evaluated by CT typically should include a brain examination as well.

An MRI can be useful in detecting morphologic alterations causing classic post-traumatic syndromes. Shear injury (the stretching and separation of gray and white matter interfaces) can be subtle and yet produce devastating clinical consequences. MRI can detect the subtle hemorrhage or edema in the classic zones of the brain susceptible to such injury. Also, both detection and localization of subtle extraaxial collections and evaluation of the major vessels at the base of the brain following basilar fracture can be rapidly accomplished with the combination of MRI and magnetic resonance angiography (MRA).

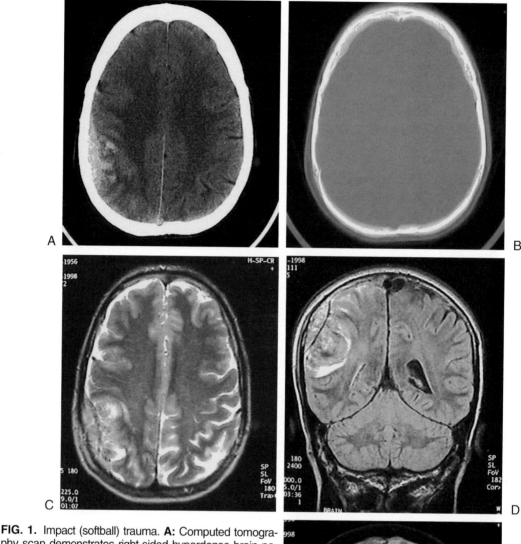

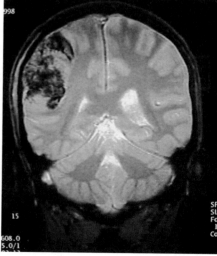

FIG. 1. Impact (softball) trauma. **A:** Computed tomography scan demonstrates right-sided hyperdense brain parenchyma and possibly extraaxial collection consistent with subdural or epidural hematoma. **B:** Bone windows demonstrate parietal skull fracture adjacent to the brain injury. **C:** T2-weighted axial (fast spin echo) study shows heterogeneous signal intensity change within the brain and inwardly convex curvilinear collection in the extraaxial space consistent with parenchymal and epidural bleeding, respectively. **D:** Coronal fluid attenuated inversion recovery (FLAIR) sequence demonstrates the heterogeneous high and low signal intensity of the parenchymal hematoma as well as the inwardly convex dural reflection containing the epidural hematoma. **E:** Gradient-recalled coronal sequence shows the dramatically lowered signal intensity of the parenchymal hematoma caused by the magnetic susceptibility effects of deoxyhemoglobin. The altered magnetic homogeneity of the bloody collection obscures the detail of the dural invagination.

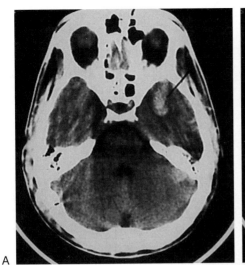
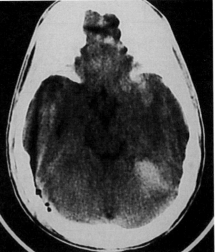

A

B

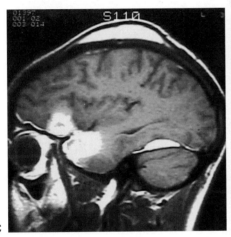

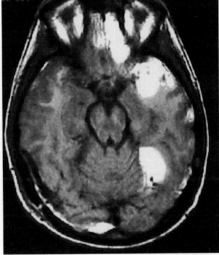

C

D

FIG. 2. Contracoup contusion. **A** and **B:** Computed tomography scans demonstrate the presence of a right occipital skull fracture, with evidence of intracranial air. Note hemorrhagic contusions of the low frontal and left temporal lobe (above the orbital roofs and adjacent to the pterion), as well as right temporal hemorrhage. Left tentorial blood collection is also shown. **C** and **D:** T1-weighted sagittal and axial sequences demonstrate the left-sided hematomas to good advantage. **E:** Coronal study shows again the contused, hemorrhagic brain above the jagged orbital roof and adjacent to the pterion. The olfactory region is involved.

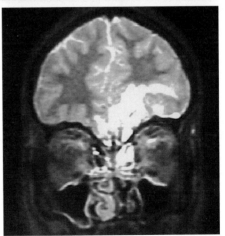

E

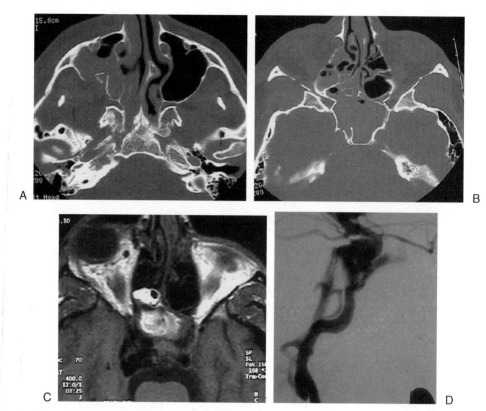

FIG. 3. Tripod fracture, skull base (sphenoid) fracture, and traumatic cavernous-carotid fistula. **A** and **B:** High-resolution computed tomography study demonstrates the components of the tripod fracture (orbital rim, zygomatic arch, and diastasis at the frontal-zygomatic suture in the lateral wall of the orbit). Note the fragmentation of the maxillary antral walls. **C:** Axial T1-weighted magnetic resonance image demonstrates prominent vessels in the region of the cavernous sinus, as well as in the right orbit behind the globe. Note proptosis. Higher slices showed an enlarged superior ophthalmic vein. Blood in the sphenoid sinuses is present as well. **D:** Selected frame from lateral right carotid angiogram verifies the presence of a traumatic cavernous-carotid fistula. Note also the dissection of the high cervical carotid artery, subpetrous segment.

III. TECHNIQUE

A. Computed Tomography

Routine brain scanning after head trauma typically includes acquisition of relatively thin sections through the posterior fossa and temporal lobes (3 to 5 mm), followed by somewhat thicker sections above the petrous ridges (7 to 10 mm). Bone windows as well as routine soft tissue windows should be filmed. When clinical signs of basilar skull fracture are present (see earlier), or when specific findings (such as hearing loss, optic nerve dysfunction, CSF leak) are present, thin slices (1 to 1.5 mm) with a bone high-resolution algorithm should be obtained through the skull base, temporal bone, or optic foramen, depending on the clinical setting. A CSF leak can be localized further by use of intrathecal injection of nonionic contrast, typically 3 to 5 mL. The dye is then brought to the intracranial space from the lumbar injection site by placing the patient in a head-down position for several minutes, and scanned, while prone. This fills the basal cisterns and demonstrates leakage of the intrathecal dye from the intracranial space through the defect typically into the paranasal sinuses, or occasionally into the middle ear or mastoid regions, depending on the site of fracture. Simultaneous injection of radioactive agents into the subarachnoid space with placement of pledgets in the nasal cavities to be counted later can be done to supplement the CT examination, but this is rarely necessary for confirmation of such leaks.

The use of ionized intravenous contrast agents is seldom necessary in the evaluation of head trauma. Modern techniques with spiral continuous scanning can be used for CT angiography and are an option for evaluating patients with basal skull trauma when vascular injury is suspected. In patients with subtle subdural fluid collection, injection of contrast can help detect the collection or characterize its cause, differentiating hematoma from inflammatory or neoplastic collections.

B. Magnetic Resonance Imaging

The typical evaluation of post-traumatic symptoms with MRI includes the acquisition of T1-weighted sagittal, T2-weighted axial, gradient-recalled (typically coronal), and fluid attenuated inversion recovery (FLAIR) images. When basal skull fracture is known to have occurred, and vascular evaluation is needed, time-of-flight MRA study of the major vessels at the skull base is undertaken. MRA can also be used to evaluate post-traumatic cervical arterial dissection.

IV. FINDINGS

Intracranial brain contusion or parenchymal hemorrhage is readily detected with routine CT technique. Hyperdense foci within the brain can be well circumscribed and solid (hematoma) or indistinct, inhomogeneous, and associated with subtle low-density zones (contusion) (see Figs. 1 and 2). Acute extraaxial collections are also readily demonstrable unless they are quite thin or occur in patients with low hematocrit levels (which reduces the CT attenuation of blood). Subdural collections typically are crescentic, conforming to the contour of the cranium's inner table. They may extend into the interhemis-

pheric or tentorial subdural space. Acute epidural collections tend to have a more lenticular morphology, inwardly convex, because they are limited from spread by the densely adherent outer dura interposed between the epidural bleed and the brain surface (see Figs. 1 and 4–9). The presence of a fluid–fluid level (hematocrit effect) can be seen occasionally in recent intracranial hematomas (see Fig. 5), the dependent red cell component particularly hyperdense on CT, with the supernatant serum showing the lower density. The mass effect of both intra- and extraaxial hematomas can vary, depending on location and on the preexisting volumetric relationships between the brain and the skull. In older individuals with an element of atrophy, as well as children in whom cranial growth has exceeded the growth rate of the brain, extraaxial accumulations can be accommodated (particularly when small) and only subsequent bleeds into the preexisting collections will produce significant mass effect (see Figs. 7 and 8). Such delayed rebleeding is not unusual in subdural hematomas, leading to a heterogeneous collection showing both low-density (old blood) and high-density (recent blood) collections.

Indeed, rebleeding even in the brain parenchyma is a known consequence of significant head injury. Delayed bleeds can occur in up to 20% of severely traumatized individuals necessitating repeat scanning particularly when clinical symptomatology is considerably worse than the initial CT predicted.

Detection of fractures is relatively straightforward, being seen as linear or jagged lucencies in the cranial vault (see Fig. 1). Thin-section, high-resolution technique aids detection of subtle fractures, particularly in the skull base (see Fig. 3). Clues to the presence of basilar fracture on the CT scan itself include opacification of the paranasal sinuses, opacification of the mastoid air cells, and the detection of intracranial air close to the skull base in the extraaxial space. Certain locations of fractures are particularly important. Fractures in the sphenoid bone and close to or crossing the cavernous sinus or carotid canal (these predispose to traumatic carotid pseudoaneurysm or formation of cavernous-carotid fistula), fractures that cross the petrous

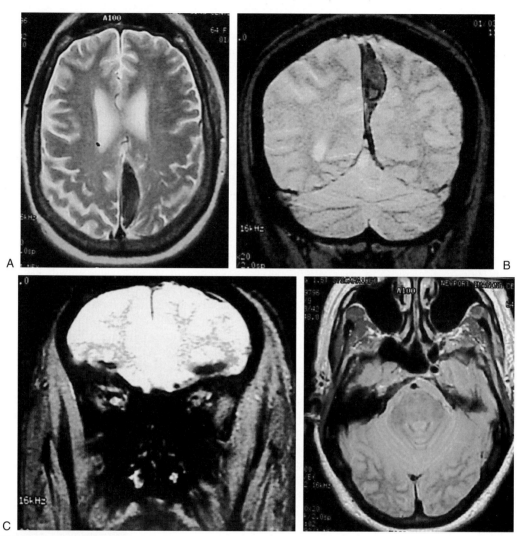

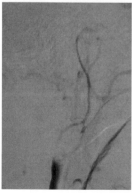

FIG. 4. Interhemispheric subdural, carotid dissection. Two weeks after a motor vehicle accident, patient presented with left leg weakness. **A:** T2-weighted axial magnetic resonance image demonstrates the blood collection in the posterior interhemispheric fissure with low signal intensity. **B** and **C:** Coronal gradient-recalled sequence documented to better advantage the interhemispheric subdural blood collection. Note the artifact of magnetic susceptibility distortion in the low frontal lobes, simulating low frontal brain contusion. No blood or edema was shown here on spin echo images. **D:** Axial "proton density" image shows absence of signal void in right cavernous carotid artery, suggesting occlusion. Punctate high signal focus is noted, suggesting perhaps a slight amount of flow within it. **E:** Late frame from a digital subtraction angiogram of the right carotid demonstrates the "string sign" of near-occlusion, due to dissection.

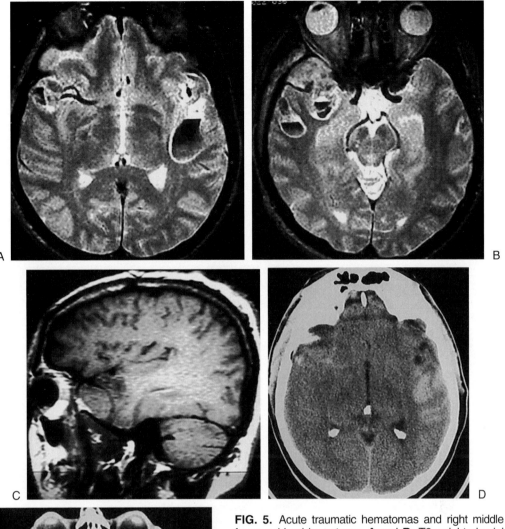

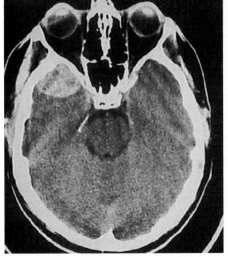

FIG. 5. Acute traumatic hematomas and right middle fossa epidural hematoma. **A** and **B:** T2-weighted axial sequences demonstrate a large hematoma in the left temporal lobe (above the petrous ridge) with fluid–fluid level of the red blood cell sediment versus serum (hematocrit effect). Note that the right temporal hematomas are smaller but also contain fluid–fluid levels. The heterogeneous collection in the anterior aspect of the right middle fossa displaces a pial vein (the curvilinear low signal structure). **C:** A T1-weighted sagittal image through the right temporal lobe verifies the presence of an epidural hematoma invaginating the right temporal pole. **D** and **E:** Accompanying computed tomography (CT) scans from the same day demonstrate the epidural blood of the right middle fossa to better advantage, but they suggest only hemorrhagic contusion of the brain as opposed to defining the frank hematomas shown by magnetic resonance imaging (MRI). Note the hyperdense epidural on CT corresponding to the isointense collection there on MRI.

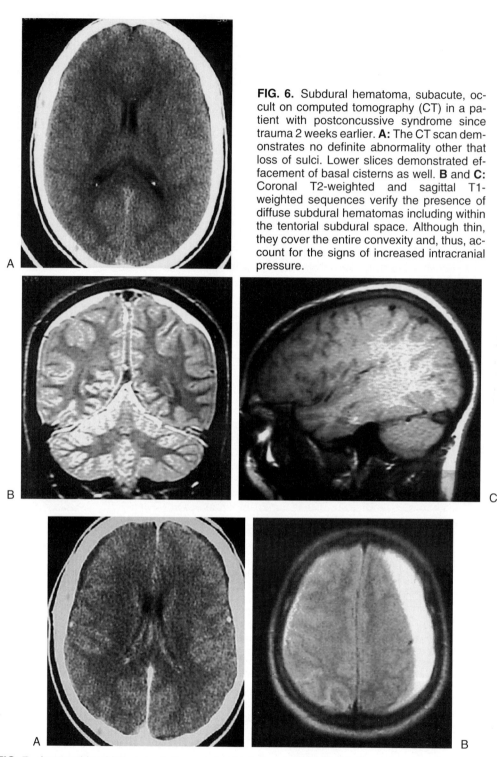

FIG. 6. Subdural hematoma, subacute, occult on computed tomography (CT) in a patient with postconcussive syndrome since trauma 2 weeks earlier. **A:** The CT scan demonstrates no definite abnormality other that loss of sulci. Lower slices demonstrated effacement of basal cisterns as well. **B** and **C:** Coronal T2-weighted and sagittal T1-weighted sequences verify the presence of diffuse subdural hematomas including within the tentorial subdural space. Although thin, they cover the entire convexity and, thus, account for the signs of increased intracranial pressure.

FIG. 7. Acute rebleed into preexisting subdural hygroma. **A:** Patient with postconcussive syndrome demonstrates small bilateral subdural hygromas on the admission computed tomography (CT) study. Patient then signed out against medical advice. **B:** A magnetic resonance image was obtained the next day, when patient returned hemiplegic after a game of squash. A T2-weighted axial image demonstrates a new left subdural hematoma, due to rebleeding.

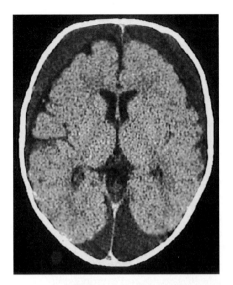

FIG. 8. Subdural hygromas of infancy. A computed tomography (CT) scan demonstrates large low-density collections surrounding the cerebral hemispheres. Although small subdural effusions can be seen as a normal variant in infants, these collections are somewhat large for the "benign subdural effusion of infancy" and demonstrate effacement of sulci as well. The brain appears relatively shrunken. Suspicion regarding occult trauma or "nonaccidental trauma" was raised given the picture.

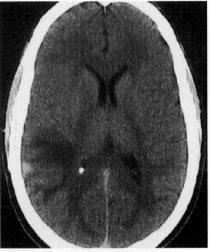

A

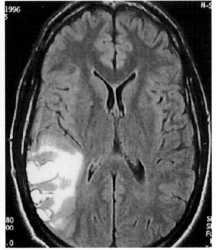

B

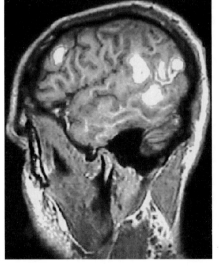

C

FIG. 9. Occult head trauma. A: Computed tomography (CT) scan of a 29-year-old man with confusion and lethargy demonstrated vague low density in the temporal white matter with suggestion of a small high-density focus just deep to the inner table. B: Axial FLAIR magnetic resonance image (MRI) shows focal collections of blood in the cortex and subcortical white matter, with vasogenic edema. C: T1-weighted sagittal image verifies the focal hemorrhagic contusions of the temporal lobe. The patient was subsequently able to give the history of having his "head kicked in" in a barroom brawl. This case demonstrates how confusing CT can be in the subacute stage of head trauma when blood density dissipates. MRI can be useful in this regard.

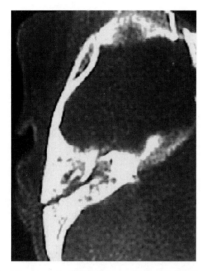

FIG. 10. Longitudinal temporal bone fracture. A computed tomography slice at the temporal bone level, bone windows, demonstrates a longitudinal fracture crossing the roof of the middle ear cavity. Conductive hearing loss was present.

bone (Fig. 10) either in the transverse or longitudinal orientation (such fractures predispose to hearing loss, which can be sensorineural when crossing the internal auditory canal, or conductive when affecting the middle ear ossicles), fractures that communicate the paranasal sinuses with the intracranial space (these necessitate prophylactic treatment for meningitis, or occasional intracranial patching with muscle or dural tissue), and fractures that cross the attachment of the major dural sinuses, or the course of the meningeal vessels (''red flags'' for the development of epidural or subdural hematoma or, occasionally, for subsequent development of sinus thrombosis or even dural or intravenous fistula) are all important to identify.

Shear injury occurs from rotational acceleration or deceleration forces producing separation of the disparately dense gray and white matter (Figs. 11 and 12). Axonal stretching and tearing, accompanied by microvascular rupture, leads to foci of hemorrhage and edema at these sites. Such forces also tend to produce contusions of the brain classically in the collicular region of the midbrain, where the rigid tentorial incisura has an impact on the brain stem. Corpus callosum may also be a site of such impact injury against the undersurface of the falx with significant rotational forces. MRI is particularly well suited for the detection of such subtle foci of injury, as well as detection of contusions along the undersurface of the brain (subfrontal and subtemporal brain surfaces are regions prone to partial-volume artifact and obscuration from streak artifact on CT scanning).

The delayed sequelae of acute head injury include infarction caused by mass effect, compression of nearby vascular beds, or compromise of the major intracranial vessels due to shifts under the falx or around the incisura. Indeed, over 90% of people who die following head injury demonstrate foci of cerebral infarction at autopsy (Fig. 13).

V. SENSITIVITY AND SPECIFICITY

Little published data exist regarding the sensitivity and specificity capabilities of CT and MRI in the setting of head trauma. The lack of a gold standard (predominately caused by the dearth of autopsy data in recent years since the introduction of these modalities) precludes definitive statistical analysis in this area. Nevertheless, it is generally accepted that CT has relatively high

FIG. 11. Shear injury in 2-year-old girl with head trauma sustained in a motor vehicle accident. **A** and **B:** Selected computed tomography (CT) slices demonstrate a subtle focal high density at the gray-white junction of the left parietal cortex, as well as a more diffuse, vague, high-density lesion in the gray-white junction of the occipital-parietal zone. **C:** T1-weighted axial study demonstrates the hemorrhagic nature of the left parietal-occipital lesion. The methemoglobin effect accounts for the bright signal on the T1-weighted image. **D** and **E:** Coronal gradient-recalled selected images demonstrate foci of low signal consistent with deoxyhemoglobin or hemosiderin at the gray-white junction. Numerous such foci were seen on the entire study. **F:** CT scan from another patient with rotational head injury demonstrates focal hemorrhage in the pontine tectum, another classic location for shear injury.

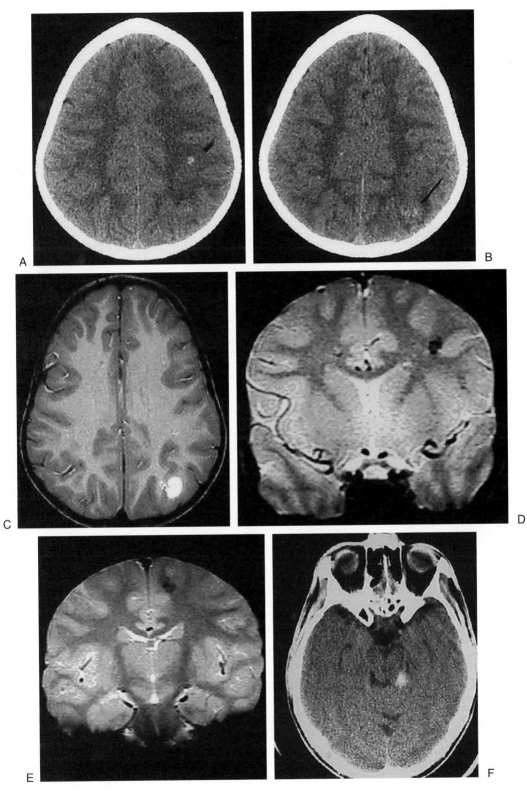

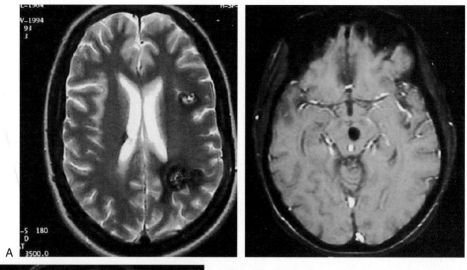

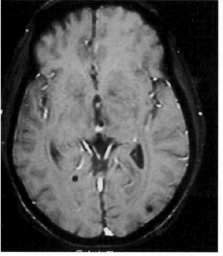

FIG. 12. Focal hemorrhagic lesions simulating shear injury. **A:** Patient has multifocal occult arteriovenous malformations, three of which are demonstrated on this T2-weighted axial image. Note the heterogeneous signal with central high intensity and the less sharply demarcated borders of the larger lesions. **B** and **C:** Patient, aged 39, had previous whole-brain radiation for lymphoma. Note focal low signal changes on these gradient-recalled axial sequences in the brain stem and subcortical junctional zones of the left occipital and posterior right temporal region, simulating shear injury. Numerous other lesions were seen as well. These are histologically correlated with capillary angioma-like change, presumably due to occlusive disease of the microvasculature caused by the radiation. Such occlusive change at the microvascular (venous) level may be the pathophysiology behind development of idiopathic occult arteriovenous malformations as well.

sensitivity for intracranial brain injury, except for axonal shear injury, and that all but the most subtle skull fractures can be detected.

VI. DIFFERENTIAL DIAGNOSIS

Given the clinical setting of head trauma, differential diagnosis for abnormalities found on CT or MRI is limited. However, occasionally patients have neurologic events that lead at least to superficial head trauma. Thus, syncopal episodes or other neurologic events that occur during such activities as driving can cause confusion between the primary and secondary causes of the subsequent morphologic abnormality found. A hypertensive bleed, for instance, can cause a patient to fall to the ground, striking his or her head, thus simulating an intracranial traumatic hemorrhage. Subarachnoid hemorrhage, almost ubiquitous in the setting of head trauma, can be due to a ruptured intracranial aneurysm, which leads to the car accident for which the patient is subsequently admitted to the emergency department suspected of having suffered head trauma during the accident. If no other cranial signs of head trauma are found on the CT, except for the subarachnoid blood, the possibility of aneurysm rupture should be considered despite the initial clinical diagnosis based on minor scalp contusions related to the

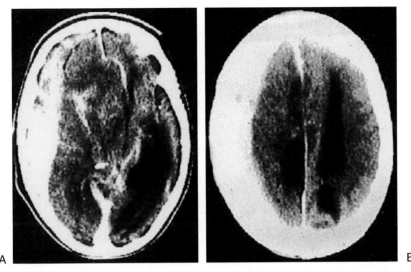

FIG. 13. Subdural hematoma, subfalcine herniation, infarction. **A** and **B:** Selected computed tomography slices demonstrate a very large right-sided subdural hematoma with herniation of the right hemisphere under the falx (note midline shift, effacement of superior cerebellar cisterns, and entrapment of the left temporal horn). Infarcts in the distribution of the left posterior cerebral artery (trapped against the free edge of the falx) and in the distribution of the anterior cerebral artery on the right (compressed against the inferior edge of the falx) are also shown.

bleed-induced fall. Occasionally, even subdural hematomas can be caused by such aneurysmal rupture. Other causes of hemorrhagic stroke (see Chapter 2) can be misdiagnosed as traumatic lesions when found in patients who are injured after the stroke-inciting event.

VII. PITFALLS

Pitfalls in the evaluation of patients with head trauma relate predominately to the limitations of the imaging modalities used. The posterior fossa is a particular problem for CT, given the presence of streak artifacts and beam-hardening artifacts in this small compartment confined predominately by bone and the rigid tentorium. Subtle collections or mass effect in this region can produce drastic clinical consequences by compromise of brain stem function. The relatively spherical bony compartment predisposes to considerable partial-volume artifact. These problems lead to difficulties with diagnosis of subtle extraaxial blood collections. Thus, particular attention to the size and location of the fourth ventricle, and any deviation of this structure from the midline, should be viewed with considerable suspicion. The morphology of the

basal cisterns should be evaluated for symmetry and preservation of typical density and size parameters.

Because certain conditions can produce extraaxial blood collections that are the same density as that of brain, subtle asymmetry of sulcal size between one cerebral convexity and the other, subtle mass effect and straightening of the typically convex junction between the gray and the white matter, and even the use of intravenous contrast for detection of such subtle isodense subdurals must be remembered. Particularly in children, there may be a normal exaggeration of the CSF space around the cerebral convexities, which arises from the disproportionate growth of the cranium and the underlying brain. Differentiation of such normal CSF prominence from old or even subacute subdural hematomas can be difficult by CT alone. MRI can readily distinguish residual blood products within such collections and can be used in supplementary fashion in suspected cases. Children also have more patent sutures at the skull base, necessitating knowledge of developmental anatomy and variation to distinguish normal structure from fractures.

VIII. SUGGESTED READINGS

Adams JH, Mitchell DE, Graham DI, Doyle D. Diffuse brain damage of immediate impact type—its relationship to 'primary brain-stem damage' in head injury. *Brain* 1977; 100:489–502.

Baker SR, Gaylord GM, Lantos G, Tabaddor K, Gallagher EJ. Emergency skull radiography: the effect of restrictive criteria on skull radiography and CT use. *Radiology* 1985; 156:409–413.

Clifton GL, Grossman RG, Makela ME, Miner ME, Handel S, Sadhu V. Neurological course and correlated computerized tomography findings after severe closed head injury. *J Neurosurg* 1980;52:611–624.

Gentry LR, Godersky JC, Thompson B, Dunn VD. Prospective comparative study of intermediate-field MR and CT in the evaluation of closed head trauma. *AJNR Am J Neuroradiol* 1988;9:91–100.

Mittl RL Jr, Grossman RI, Hiehle JF Jr, et al. Prevalence of MR evidence of diffuse axonal injury in patients with mild head injury and normal head CT findings. *AJNR Am J Neuroradiol* 1994;15:1583–1589.

2

Stroke

Michael Brant-Zawadzki

I. CLINICAL OVERVIEW

More than 500,000 Americans suffer a stroke annually, making it the most common single indication for emergency cross-sectional imaging of the brain. Unfortunately, the term "stroke" is nonspecific. It is used for any sudden intracranial event that leads to a permanent neurologic deficit. Causes of stroke include infarction, anoxia, carbon monoxide poisoning, drug ingestion and its effects, seizure, hemorrhage caused by hypertension or amyloid angiopathy, venous thrombosis, aneurysmal or arteriovenous malformation rupture, bleeding from iatrogenic causes or a natural diathesis, spontaneous subdural hematoma, and bleeding into a tumor. Obviously, cross-sectional imaging is an important tool in triage of patients to appropriate therapy.

Hyperacute ischemic insults may be potentially reversible with thrombolytic therapy, which would be contraindicated in the hemorrhagic entities causing stroke. In addition, the blood vessels leading to the brain should be evaluated because invasive interventions, such as intraarterial thrombolytic therapy and even endarterectomy in certain cases, may be useful in the earliest stages of ischemia. Finally, more than 30% of patients who present with a transient ischemic event and recover clinically within 24 hours harbor frank cerebral infarction. Because such infarcts preclude surgical therapy for the first several weeks, cross-sectional imaging is necessary even in patients who have no permanent neurologic residual and are being consid-ered for carotid endarterectomy after a transient ischemic attack.

II. IMAGING STRATEGY

Most protocols for acute stroke choose computed tomography (CT) as the primary imaging method in the earliest stages because of its ready availability and rapid imaging capability, as well as its ability to separate ischemic from hemorrhagic strokes. However, a strong argument is emerging that magnetic resonance imaging (MRI) combined with magnetic resonance angiography (MRA) should replace CT. This argument rests on the ability of MRI to more sensitively identify ischemic infarction as compared to CT and also its ability to evaluate the vessels leading to the brain at the same sitting (Fig. 1). The detection of acute hemorrhage is also sensitive with MRI (see later). The need to identify reversible stages of cerebral ischemia appears to be better met by MRI than CT in experimental models as well as in early clinical experience with new MRI techniques. Therefore, when patients present within the first 6 hours of stroke, and are able to undergo MRI (some degree of cooperation, absence of implanted pacemakers, no need for life support systems being the main criteria), the combination of modern MRI/MRA may well be replacing CT as the modality of choice in the first 6 hours. After that time frame, MRI still has the advantage although presentation of stroke after 6 hours allows for relatively little in the way of beneficial patient manage-

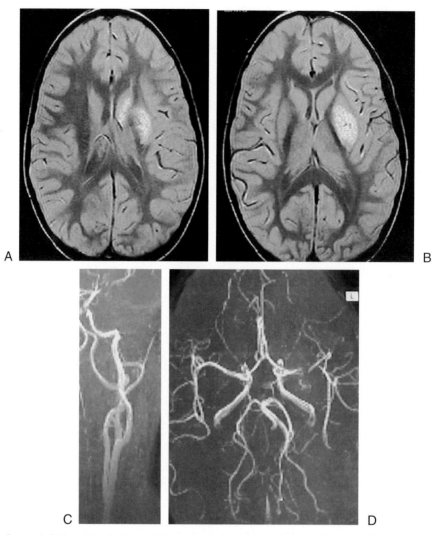

FIG. 1. Acute right hemiplegia in a child, aged 5, transferred from outlying facility for angiography. **A** and **B:** T2-weighted, first echo images demonstrate infarcts of the lenticular nucleus and caudate head (corpus striatum), seen as high signal lesions within these gray matter structures. **C** and **D:** Carotid and intracranial magnetic resonance angiography (MRA) demonstrates a normal left cervical carotid artery, but a filling defect in the left middle cerebral artery consistent with clot is shown. Patent foramen ovale was subsequently found. The combined magnetic resonance imaging/MRA study obviated an invasive cerebral arteriogram in this child.

ment and CT suffices for establishing the cause in the vast majority of strokes.

III. TECHNIQUE

The choice of modality to evaluate acute stroke is dictated by the availability of aggressive therapeutic methodologies for acute ischemia in a given clinical setting. If an interventional endovascular team is available, and intraarterial thrombolytic therapy is a consideration in the first few hours, MRI offers considerable advantages because it can identify hyperacute ischemia, which may be reversible by using a combination of diffusion and conventional imaging. Diffusion images take less than a minute or two to obtain. T1-weighted sagittal, late echo T2-weighted axial, fluid attenuated inversion recovery (FLAIR) axial sequences, and gradient-recalled coronal sequences can all be performed in 20 minutes or less with modern high-field equipment. The combination of MRI/MRA can detect middle cerebral artery occlusive disease when present and also clear the pathway for a catheter technique in the cervical carotid. Perfusion imaging in combination with diffusion imaging may well be the ultimate triage methodology for determining which patients undergo intraarterial thrombolysis. Perfusion imaging currently can be performed with intravenous injection of paramagnetic contrast, a large perfusion defect in the face of a small or absent diffusion (as well as conventional spin echo) abnormality being a strong indicator for possible reversal of ischemia with thrombolytic therapy.

When CT is used, thin-section technique in the posterior fossa (3 to 5 mm) and conventional slice thickness (7 to 10 mm) in the supratentorial compartment should be used. Intravenous contrast enhancement should be avoided in the acute setting because large boluses of iodinated intravenous contrast can alter hemodynamics (including production of hypotension) and may be potentially neurotoxic in the face of a broken blood–brain barrier, although this is controversial.

IV. FINDINGS

The findings on cross-sectional imaging in the setting of stroke can be divided on the basis of ischemic versus hemorrhagic entities. Infarction typically involves gray matter predominately because of its high metabolic rate producing preferential vulnerability to ischemia. In general, a single vascular territory of the gray matter cortical mantle demonstrates altered signal intensity on MRI or lower density on CT.

A CT scan may demonstrate asymmetric high density in the proximal middle cerebral artery trunk in patients with embolic infarction. MRA demonstrates an asymmetric decrease in vasculature in the involved territory in such patients, if not frank occlusion of the proximal middle cerebral artery trunk. Little mass effect is seen in the first 24 hours of infarction. Thus, subtle effacement of sulci may be the only finding indicating volume change. An MRI more readily shows the altered brain's increased signal intensity on T2-weighted images as compared to CT demonstration of low attenuation in the involved region (Fig. 2). If intravenous contrast is used on MRI, slowed flow shows enhancement by gadolinium and is an early sign of ischemia (Fig. 3). Subtle loss of gray-white density difference on CT and an obscured outline of the lentiform nucleus, loss of the density of the insular ribbon, can be additional clues on the CT scan. Decisions critical to the triage of patients for intravenous thrombolytic and even coagulant therapy in the first few hours after infarction rest on the amount of middle cerebral territory involved by such subtle ischemic changes. Large territorial ischemia (more than 33%) contraindicates such therapy. MRI makes management decisions easier because of better discrimination of ischemia, particularly when diffusion imaging is used (Figs. 4 and 5). Anoxic insults typically produce changes in the basal ganglia as well as in the cortical ribbon diffusely throughout the brain, as opposed to a single vascular territory (Fig. 6). Watershed infarcts demonstrate a distinct geography, the border zones of the brain between two vascular territories demonstrating the signal or density alteration, starting at the cortical mantle and extending into the deep white matter watershed of the centrum semiovale (Fig. 7).

An MRI can detect acute hemorrhage, the gra-

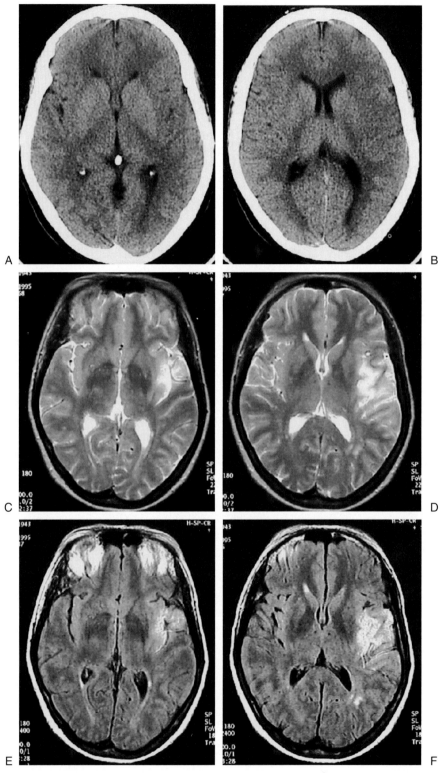

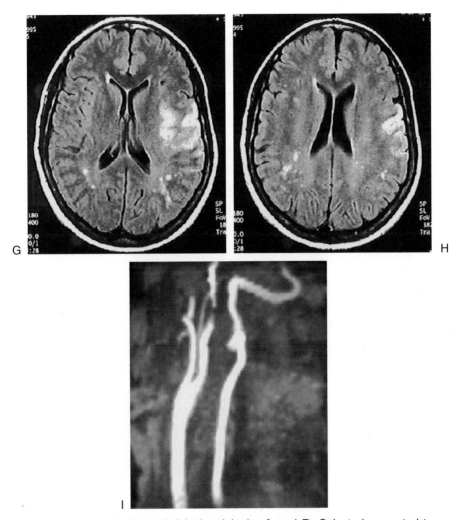

FIG. 2. Acute onset of aphasia and right hemiplegia. **A** and **B:** Selected computed tomographic slices obtained 4 hours after onset demonstrate very subtle loss of gray matter density in the left insula and subtle loss of gray-white matter differentiation in the opercular cortex. Note asymmetry of sulci, the left being less visible than the right. This was also noted on the next higher slice. **C** and **D:** T2-weighted (second echo) images verify high signal intensity in the insular and temporal lobe cortex. Note sparing of white matter. Note signal void is present within some middle cerebral artery branches. **E–H:** FLAIR images show to better advantage the involvement of the gray matter, as the high signal from cerebrospinal fluid seen on the T2-weighted images is suppressed with the FLAIR sequence. Again note white matter sparing. Incidentally, microangiopathic white matter lesions are seen elsewhere. **I:** Selected frame from magnetic resonance angiogram depicts midcervical internal carotid artery dissection as the cause for the embolic infarct.

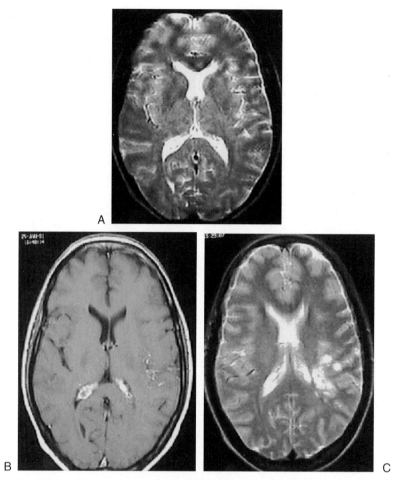

FIG. 3. Acute ischemia, 4 hours of aphasia, and right hemiparesis. **A:** T2-weighted axial image demonstrates no obvious abnormality on the acute study. Note asymmetry of signal void; the left distal middle cerebral branches are not seen as compared to the right side. **B:** Scan obtained after intravenous contrast injection demonstrates enhancement of posterior sylvian vessels. **C:** Scan obtained 24 hours after the initial study shows infarction in the posterior middle cerebral artery distribution served by the enhancing vessels.

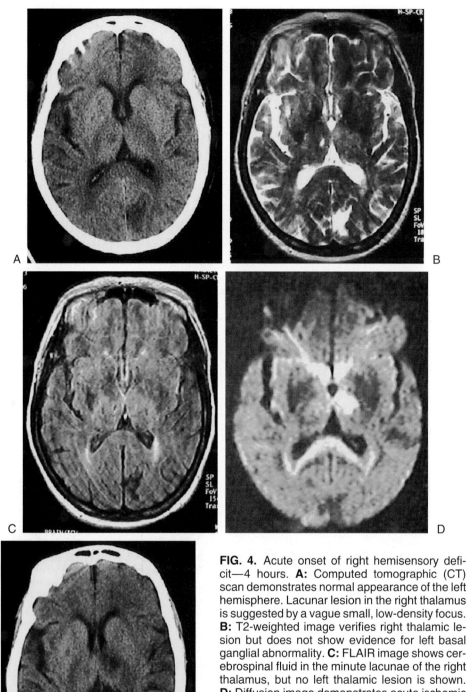

FIG. 4. Acute onset of right hemisensory deficit—4 hours. **A:** Computed tomographic (CT) scan demonstrates normal appearance of the left hemisphere. Lacunar lesion in the right thalamus is suggested by a vague small, low-density focus. **B:** T2-weighted image verifies right thalamic lesion but does not show evidence for left basal ganglial abnormality. **C:** FLAIR image shows cerebrospinal fluid in the minute lacunae of the right thalamus, but no left thalamic lesion is shown. **D:** Diffusion image demonstrates acute ischemic change in the left thalamus, the right showing no signal changes. This accounts for the acute onset of the new right hemisensory change in the patient. **E:** The CT scan 24 hours after magnetic resonance imaging now shows the new left thalamic infarction. Diffusion is the most sensitive method for evaluating ischemia. Note old left occipital infarct (**A–C**).

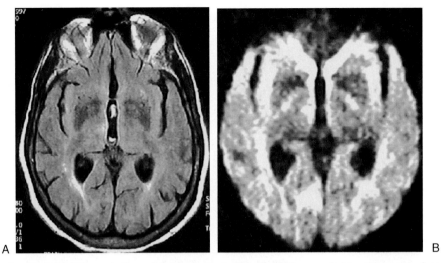

FIG. 5. Acute onset (3 hours) of quadrantanopsia **A:** The FLAIR image demonstrates no abnormality in the occipital or calcarine cortex. Scattered punctate microangiopathic changes are seen. The other conventional magnetic resonance imaging sequences were negative other than for diffuse microangiopathic disease. **B:** Diffusion image demonstrates a small zone of high signal in the right calcarine cortex, accounting for the left quadrantanopsia.

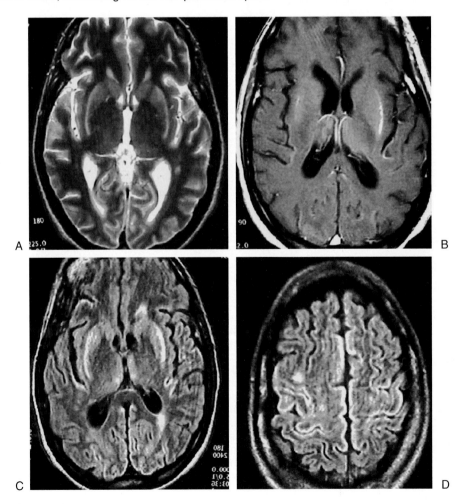

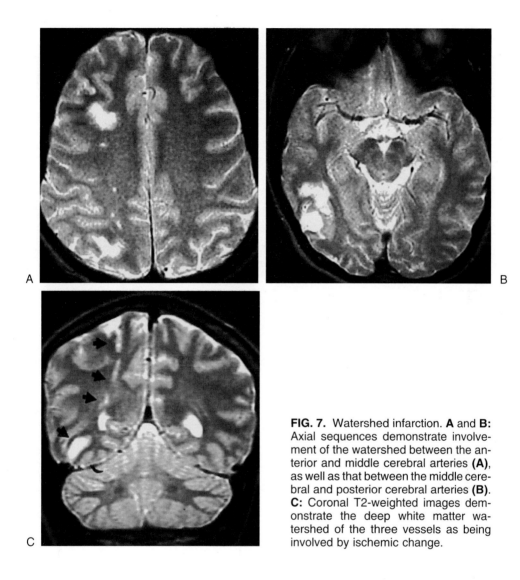

FIG. 7. Watershed infarction. **A** and **B:** Axial sequences demonstrate involvement of the watershed between the anterior and middle cerebral arteries **(A)**, as well as that between the middle cerebral and posterior cerebral arteries **(B)**. **C:** Coronal T2-weighted images demonstrate the deep white matter watershed of the three vessels as being involved by ischemic change.

FIG. 6. Diffuse anoxia in 32-year-old woman with cardiorespiratory arrest after overdose with narcotic. **A:** T2-weighted image at the level of the basal ganglia demonstrates subtle increased signal intensity of the lenticular nuclei and caudate nuclear head. **B:** Curvilinear enhancement of the lenticular nuclei is noted on the T1-weighted postcontrast image. **C** and **D:** FLAIR sequence demonstrates the increased signal of the lenticular nuclei, as well as the cortical ribbon in the posterior insular region (*left*) and in the convexity and parasagittal gray matter.

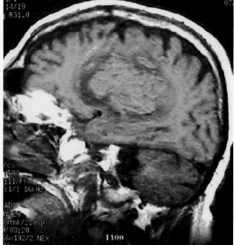

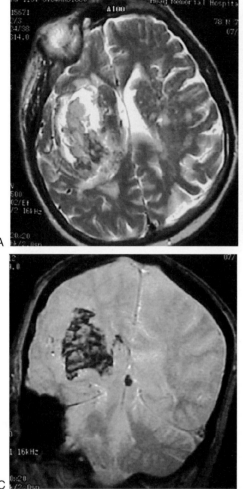

FIG. 8. Hypertensive basal ganglial hemorrhage. **A:** T2-weighted axial study at 3 hours after the stroke demonstrates large heterogeneous mass in the right basal ganglial region with mass effect. The location and presence of mass effect, as well as the heterogeneous signal, are quite atypical for acute infarction in this stroke patient. **B:** T1-weighted sagittal sequence demonstrates inhomogeneous signal in the mass as well. **C:** Gradient-recalled sequence demonstrates preferentially lowered signal intensity interspersed throughout the mass.

dient-recalled sequences being most sensitive to altered local magnetic field homogeneity and resulting low signal intensity (Figs. 8 and 9). Usually, a mass (as opposed to infarction) is seen not in a typical arterial territory, but rather deep in the brain, the signal intensity of which is heterogeneous with low signal foci (due to deoxyhemoglobin) particularly present (Fig. 10). A fluid–fluid level can sometimes be seen in acute hematomas due to the hematocrit effect (dependent red blood cells settling by gravity, serum above). Hemorrhagic conversion of bland infarcts occurs in the second week in almost 50% of all infarcts. Infarcts of the middle cerebral artery may bleed 2 to 3 days out with acute clinical deterioration (see Fig. 9).

Intracranial hemorrhage is readily detected by CT as a zone of high density typically in the deep basal ganglia of the brain, possibly dissecting into the ventricular system, when it is hypertensive in origin. Posterior fossa location also suggests hypertensive etiology. Amyloid angiopathy has become perhaps a more common cause of intracranial hemorrhage, producing typically subcortical bleeds, with recurrences over time. Subarachnoid hemorrhage and extraaxial bleeding can also be readily identified by change of cerebrospinal fluid (CSF) density on CT, as well as the classic morphology of concave (subdural) or convex (epidural) bleeds (see Fig. 10).

If contrast material is used, gyriform enhance-

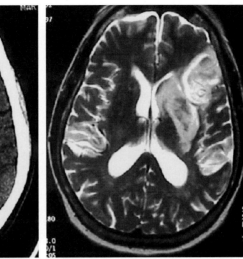

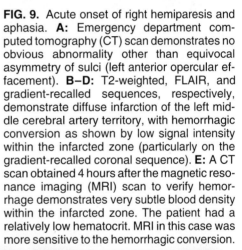

FIG. 9. Acute onset of right hemiparesis and aphasia. **A:** Emergency department computed tomography (CT) scan demonstrates no obvious abnormality other than equivocal asymmetry of sulci (left anterior opercular effacement). **B–D:** T2-weighted, FLAIR, and gradient-recalled sequences, respectively, demonstrate diffuse infarction of the left middle cerebral artery territory, with hemorrhagic conversion as shown by low signal intensity within the infarcted zone (particularly on the gradient-recalled coronal sequence). **E:** A CT scan obtained 4 hours after the magnetic resonance imaging (MRI) scan to verify hemorrhage demonstrates very subtle blood density within the infarcted zone. The patient had a relatively low hematocrit. MRI in this case was more sensitive to the hemorrhagic conversion.

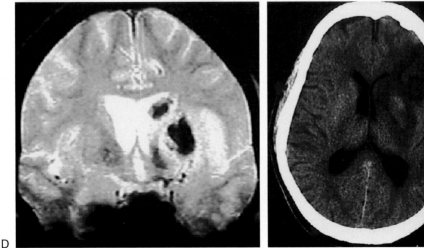

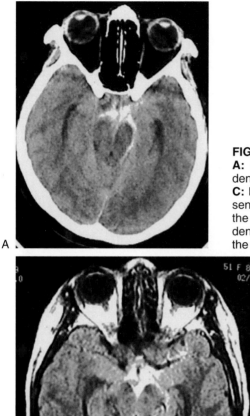

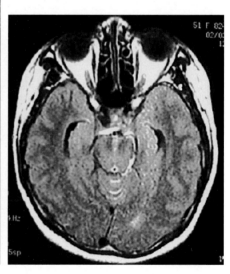

FIG. 10. Stroke from subarachnoid hemorrhage. **A:** Computed tomography demonstrates blood density in the perimesencephalic cisterns. **B** and **C:** FLAIR sequences show blood in the perimesencephalic cistern, particularly the left side, with the cerebrospinal fluid–blood level in the dependent left ventricular atrium as well. Note blood in the vermian sulci on the higher slice.

A

B

C

ment in the cortex is shown both on MRI and CT in the subacute stages of infarction. In the acute stage, MRI can show asymmetric enhancement of the vessels within which decreased flow to the brain produced the infarct (see Fig. 3).

V. SENSITIVITY AND SPECIFICITY

Sensitivity of CT scans to territorial infarcts within the 24 hours is in the 50% to 60% range, with some studies suggesting sensitivity as great as 90%, although with considerable interobserver variability. Obviously, smaller infarcts in the distribution of perforating arteries particularly in the posterior fossa and internal capsular regions are difficult to identify with CT scanning. MRI sensitivity to acute infarction, especially with use of diffusion sequences, is greater than 80%. Detection of hemorrhage is extremely sensitive with CT scanning (greater than 90%). The sensitivity rate for MRI is not yet established because its use in acute stroke and particularly acute hemorrhage has not been statistically established; however, recent articles suggest a sensitivity equal to that of CT in the detection of hemorrhage (see Fig. 9), including that in the subarachnoid space when the FLAIR sequence is used (this sequence voids the normal CSF signal, making recognition of abnormal CSF quite easy-see Fig. 10).

VI. DIFFERENTIAL DIAGNOSIS

Classical infarction involving cortex in a vascular territory has a relatively narrow differential diagnosis when the clinical onset is known. Occasionally, infection can produce an acute presentation of neurologic dysfunction and involve the cortex. Herpes encephalitis is a prime example in the adult. The temporal lobe shows alteration of signal intensity although there is typically slightly greater white matter involvement and mass effect than in acute infarction, but the clinical and imaging manifestations may simulate infarction. Small hemorrhagic foci and bilaterality will help suggest herpes (see Chapter 3). Postictal brain can

demonstrate edema in the cortex at the site of epileptiform activity and can therefore simulate infarction particularly if Todd's paralysis is clinically present in the postictal setting. Hypertensive encephalopathy as well as postpartum (or prepartum) eclampsia can produce acute neurologic change and alteration of brain cortex similar to infarction in that edema of the gray matter is shown. This most often can be seen in the occipital regions simulating bilateral posterior cerebral artery infarction due to basilar embolization (Fig. 11). The clinical history is obviously helpful in this regard. MELAS (mitochondrial encephalopathy, lactic acidosis, and seizures) syndrome can also produce lesions in the cortex similar to acute cerebral infarction (pathologically as well) (Fig. 12). Acute migraine can produce a transient strokelike presentation, with permanent deficits caused by the associated spasm occasionally resulting (Fig. 13).

VII. PITFALLS

Elderly patients with deep hemispheric focal white matter lesions are problematic when they present with acute neurologic change in that detection of the given acute event is difficult. Diffusion imaging is helpful in this regard with MRI because abnormalities on the diffusion images indicate acute change (restricted diffusion of water when shifted into the intracellular compartment), helping to separate such lesions from the gliotic, demyelinated foci of chronic microangiopathic change in the brain.

Focal brain hemorrhage should be followed with subsequent scans at 3- to 6-month intervals to ensure that what at first presentation appeared to be a spontaneous intracranial hemorrhage does not harbor a pathologic substrate such as a tumor or vascular malformation. Diffusion imaging can occasionally be falsely positive for ischemia in small-cell neoplasms (Fig. 14).

Patients who develop intracranial hemorrhage while severely anemic may not show the typical high density on CT, thus making the differential diagnosis more difficult. Also, if patients are seen in the subacute phase of a

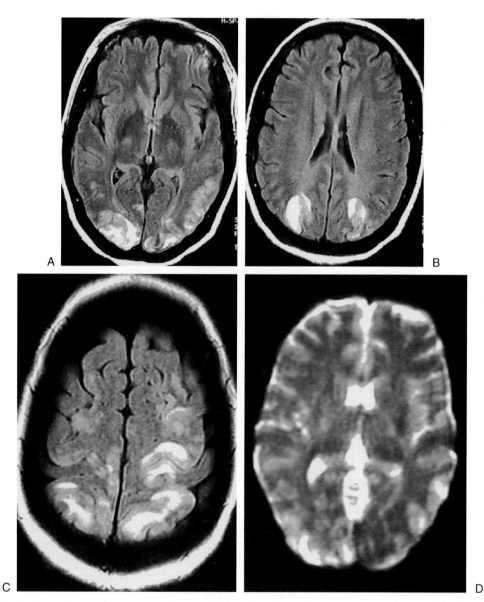

FIG. 11. Hypertensive encephalopathy in patient presenting to the emergency department with acute delirium and strokelike neurologic deficits bilaterally. **A–C:** FLAIR images demonstrate multifocal zones of altered signal intensity involving the gray and subcortical white matter. **D–F:** Diffusion sequences show less involvement. The pathophysiology of hypertensive encephalopathy includes ischemia as well as vasogenic edema, both shown well by FLAIR sequences; diffusion only shows the ischemic brain edema (due to cell swelling) as opposed to the vasogenic edema.

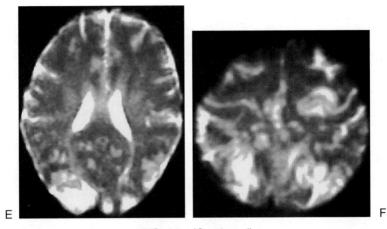

E   F

FIG. 11. *(Continued)*

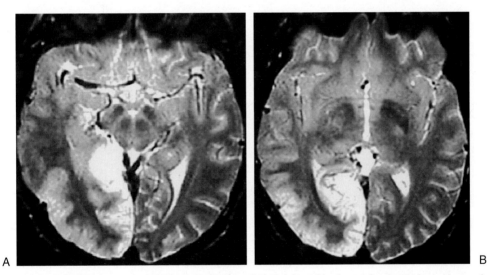

A   B

FIG. 12. The MELAS (mitochondrial encephalopathy, lactic acidosis, and seizures) syndrome in a young man presenting with seizure, left hemiparesis, and visual deficit. **A** and **B:** Selected T2-weighted images demonstrate diffuse gray matter signal alteration in the distribution of the posterior temporal and occipital territory.

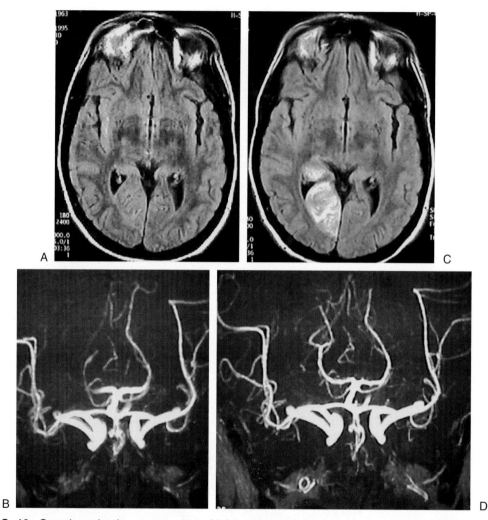

FIG. 13. Complex migraine; acute onset of left hemianopsia in a young woman with history of migraines, with an acute migraine headache accompanying the deficit. **A** and **B:** FLAIR and magnetic resonance angiography (MRA) images demonstrate no abnormality in the visual cortex. However, the right posterior cerebral artery demonstrates markedly diminished caliber consistent with spasm. **C** and **D:** FLAIR and MRA studies obtained 6 days later demonstrate a zone of infarction in the right occipital cortex. Note the posterior cerebral artery has reconstituted. The patient's symptoms were dramatically improved! The occipital lesion may represent edema only.

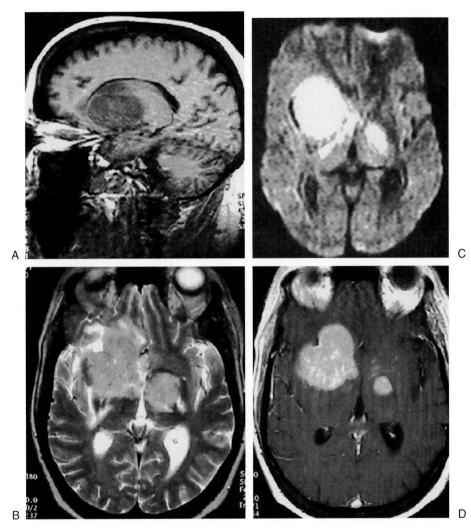

FIG. 14. Metastatic disease presenting with stroke. **A** and **B:** T1-weighted sagittal and T2-weighted axial sequences demonstrate lesions in the basal ganglia suggesting infarcts given the acute stroke presentation of this patient. **C:** Diffusion image verifies high signal intensity of the lesions as would be expected for an ischemic insult. **D:** Contrast-enhanced T1-weighted axial image demonstrates homogeneous enhancement of the lesions totally atypical for acute infarct. Metastatic melanoma was subsequently verified. Small-cell neoplasms in the brain can produce a crowded extracellular space with resulting restriction of diffusion, simulating intracellular edema of ischemic insults on diffusion images. Note that the signal intensity of the lesions on T2-weighted images is relatively isointense, atypical for infarction.

focal brain hemorrhage on CT, iso- or hypo-dense lesions in the brain may hide their original hemorrhagic nature unless an MRI scan is obtained (see Chapter 1).

VIII. SUGGESTED READINGS

Fisher M, Prichard JW, Warach S. New magnetic resonance techniques for acute ischemic stroke. *JAMA* 1995;274: 908–911.

Gomori JM, Grossman RI. Mechanisms responsible for the MR appearance and evolution of intracranial hemorrhage. *RadioGraphics* 1988;8:427–454.

Matsumura K, Matsuda M, Handa J, Todo G. Magnetic resonance imaging with aneurysmal subarachnoid hemorrhage: comparison with computed tomography scan. *Surg Neurol* 1990;34:71–80.

Von Kummer R, Allen KL, Holle R, et al. Acute stroke: usefulness of early CT findings before thrombolytic therapy. *Radiology* 1997;205:327–333.

Von Kummer R, Holle R, Grzyska U, et al. Interobserver agreement in assessing early CT signs of middle cerebral artery infarction. *AJNR Am J Neuroradiol* 1996;17: 1743–1748.

3

Fever and Neurologic Signs

Rule Out Central Nervous System Infection

Michael Brant-Zawadzki

I. CLINICAL OVERVIEW

Infection in the central nervous system (CNS) is often a consideration in patients who present to the emergency department with altered mental status and fever, although in the majority of such cases the altered mental status is the result of the constitutional illness rather than any frank brain infection. The clinical diagnosis of meningitis is frequently considered as part of the differential in patients seen for acute, severe headache. Also, the first-ever seizure in an individual who has fever or other constitutional signs raises the suspicion of CNS infection. Finally, the immunocompromised host with a new onset of focal neurologic signs may also be aggressively evaluated for CNS infection. Whereas lumbar puncture remains the gold standard for diagnosis of meningitis, cross-sectional imaging is often necessary to exclude intracranial mass before lumbar puncture and may readily identify parenchymal brain infection as well as extraaxial empyema.

II. IMAGING STRATEGY

Magnetic resonance imaging (MRI) is the best and only imaging study needed in the evaluation of patients with suspected CNS infection, although in patients who cannot undergo MRI (those with pacemakers, on life support equipment, and the like), computed tomography (CT) of the brain is certainly a viable option. The multiparametric and multiplanar capabilities of MRI allow for greater sensitivity in detecting infec-

tion as compared to CT, including the detection of meningitis and easy depiction of early cerebritis and associated abnormalities. Evaluation of the spine can also be accomplished with MRI in selected patients, when necessary, at the same sitting.

III. TECHNIQUE

An MRI screening study of the brain using T1-weighted sagittal, T2-weighted axial (dual echo) imaging is supplemented by an axial fluid attenuated inversion recovery (FLAIR) sequence as well as a set of pre- and postcontrast T1-weighted axial sequences. Magnetic resonance angiography (MRA) may be useful for patients with suspected vasculitis, although subtle mycotic aneurysms seen rarely with endocarditis require the spatial resolution of conventional angiography for detection. If MRI is not possible, conventional pre- and postcontrast CT scanning can be used instead. Typical section thickness (3 to 5 mm in the posterior fossa, 7 to 10 mm above) is used.

IV. FINDINGS

Acute meningitis, particularly when viral, is almost never seen on CT or MRI. Lumbar puncture remains the gold standard for this diagnosis. The FLAIR sequence can detect cerebrospinal fluid (CSF) that is altered by proteinaceous or other material, thus enabling the detection of acute meningitis even when contrast-enhanced

T1-weighted images do not demonstrate meningeal inflammation (Figs. 1 and 2). Such inflammation is shown more often in severe bacterial and particularly granulomatous forms of meningitis either on contrast-enhanced CT or T1-weighted images. Separation of meningeal enhancement from enhancement of the vascular space is more readily discernable on MRI, where vessels demonstrate signal void (as opposed to enhancement similar to that of the meninges on CT). Infected paranasal sinuses or temporal mastoid air cells (as well as middle ear cavities) can be a clue to infection as can the presence of hydrocephalus caused by altered CSF resorption (Fig. 3).

Parenchymal cerebritis presents early as an ill-defined smallish zone of edema typically at the gray-white matter junctional zone. Mild mass effect accompanies the findings of low density of CT or signal intensity elevation on T2-weighted MRI. This zone becomes better defined over the subsequent 3 to 4 days, developing a discrete capsule by 7 to 10 days. This capsule can be seen as a ring of high intensity on precontrast T1-weighted images, or hyperdensity on CT, which also vividly enhances after

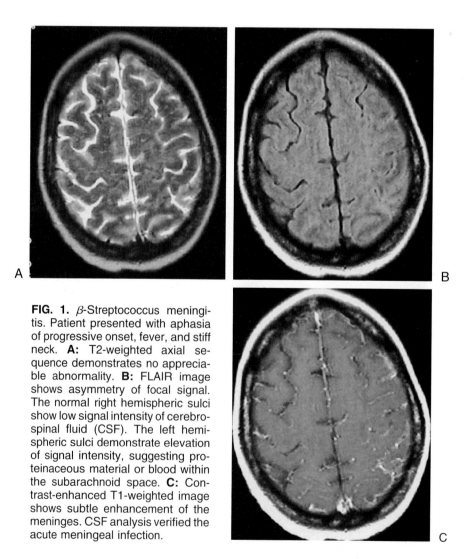

FIG. 1. β-Streptococcus meningitis. Patient presented with aphasia of progressive onset, fever, and stiff neck. **A:** T2-weighted axial sequence demonstrates no appreciable abnormality. **B:** FLAIR image shows asymmetry of focal signal. The normal right hemispheric sulci show low signal intensity of cerebrospinal fluid (CSF). The left hemispheric sulci demonstrate elevation of signal intensity, suggesting proteinaceous material or blood within the subarachnoid space. **C:** Contrast-enhanced T1-weighted image shows subtle enhancement of the meninges. CSF analysis verified the acute meningeal infection.

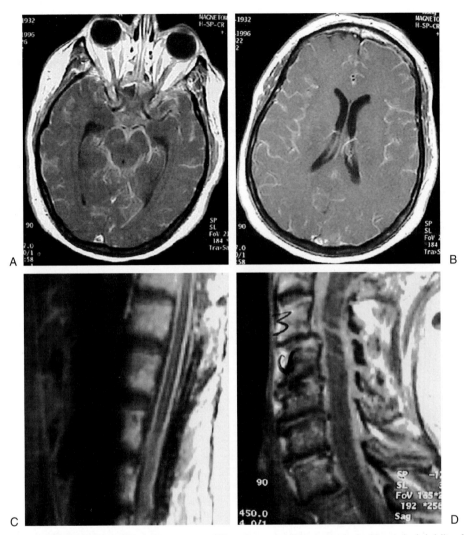

FIG. 2. Acute meningitis, subdural empyema. Woman, aged 64, presented with nuchal rigidity, fever, delirium, and leg weakness, and progressed rapidly to a semicomatose state. **A** and **B:** Selected axial magnetic resonance imaging T1-weighted postcontrast studies show diffuse enhancement of the leptomeninges in the basal cisterns and within the sulci. **C** and **D:** T1-weighted postcontrast sagittal images of the spinal canal demonstrate diffuse enhancement of the subdural space extending from the thoracic region into the cervical and prepontine subdural space. Lumbar puncture verified acute empyema and meningitis, secondary to staphylococcus. Patient had dental surgery a month previously and was subsequently found to have a hypergammaglobulinemia.

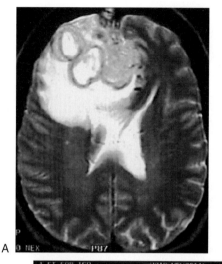

FIG. 3. Brain abscess secondary to sinusitis. **A:** A T2-weighted axial study demonstrates a considerable amount of mass effect and edema in the right frontal lobe with early extension into the contralateral hemisphere. **B** and **C:** T1-weighted sagittal pre- and postcontrast sequences demonstrate ring-enhancing lesions within the grossly abnormal right frontal lobe, with a bizarre pattern. Note opacification of the frontal sinus on all the images, the contrast enhancement bridging the dura. **D:** Axial postcontrast study shows the thick-walled abscesses. **E:** The postoperative study obtained 2 days later demonstrates considerable improvement in mass effect following debridement of the abscesses. The patient had a history of rheumatoid arthritis with chronic steroid therapy and recent sinusitis. His symptoms were surprisingly mild, a factor attributable to the chronic steroid therapy.

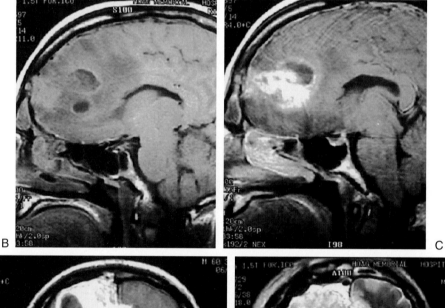

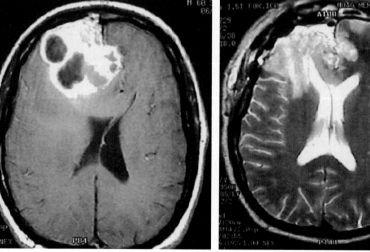

paramagnetic contrast injection both on T1-weighted MRI or CT after intravenous injection of an iodinated agent (Figs. 4 and 5). The surrounding vasogenic edema may be striking, particularly with small abscesses in which the surrounding edema seems out of proportion to the size of the lesion (due to the considerable blood–brain barrier breakdown produced by the infectious process). Focal calcification can be seen in lesions produced by cysticercosis, al-

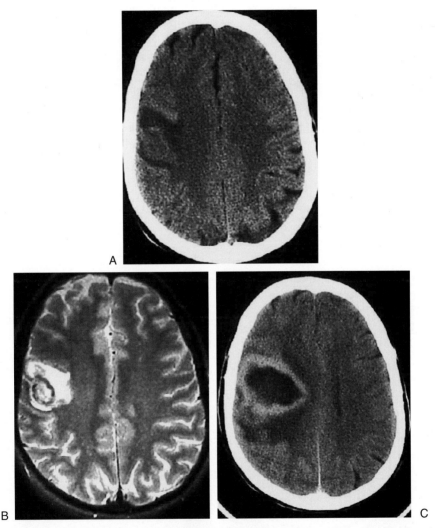

FIG. 4. Evolution of brain abscess. Woman, aged 54, presented with acute onset of left hemiparesis and confusion. **A:** Admitting computed tomography (CT) scan done in the evening demonstrates a low-density region in the right posterior frontal lobe initially interpreted as infarction. **B:** Magnetic resonance imaging (MRI) scan the next day demonstrates vasogenic edema in the right posterior frontal cortex, with subtle ring of low signal intensity within. This was thought due to hemorrhagic conversion of the infarct, although the patient's signs of fever and elevated white cell count led to lumbar puncture, which suggested infection. She was started on antibiotics. **C:** A CT scan obtained 5 days later demonstrates rapid progression of the abscess with enhancing capsule now being seen. Note thinning on the inner margin. (*Figure continues.*)

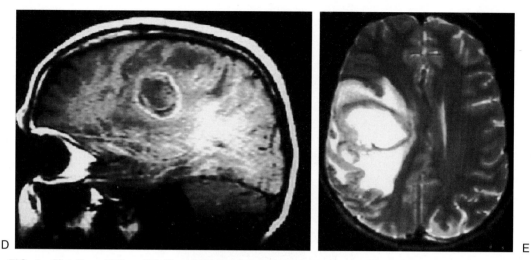

D   E

FIG. 4. *(Continued.)* **D** and **E:** The MRI later the same day demonstrates the capsule of the abscess as showing a high signal ring on T1-weighted noncontrast images; the capsule is seen as a low signal intensity ring (with thinner inner margin) on the T2-weighted axial study. The patient eventually recovered on intravenous antibiotics. She had a history of dental work approximately 3 weeks before presentation.

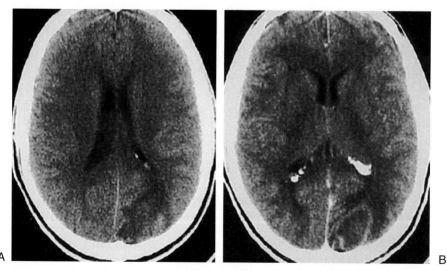

A   B

FIG. 5. Anaerobic abscess. A 35-year-old man presented with headache and mild obtundation. **A:** Admitting computed tomography (CT) scan demonstrates a diffuse low-density region of a nonspecific nature in the left occipital pole. **B:** A CT scan obtained the next morning with contrast demonstrates vague garland-shaped enhancement in the low-density region with mass effect, atypical for acute infarction given this mass effect and edema. *(Figure continues.)*

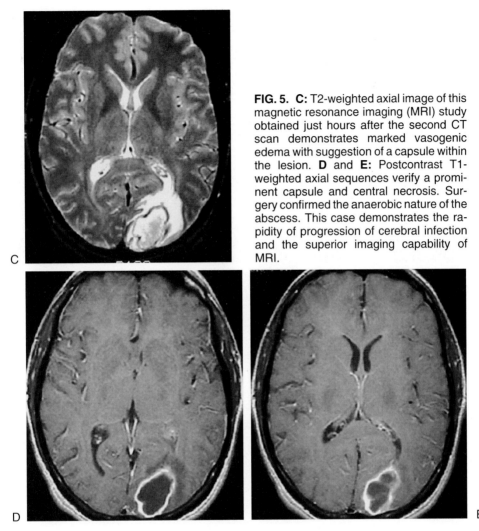

C

D

E

FIG. 5. C: T2-weighted axial image of this magnetic resonance imaging (MRI) study obtained just hours after the second CT scan demonstrates marked vasogenic edema with suggestion of a capsule within the lesion. **D** and **E:** Postcontrast T1-weighted axial sequences verify a prominent capsule and central necrosis. Surgery confirmed the anaerobic nature of the abscess. This case demonstrates the rapidity of progression of cerebral infection and the superior imaging capability of MRI.

though these patients rarely present with fever; seizure is the typical indication for scanning (Figs. 6 and 7). MRI may have difficulty in detecting such calcification unless gradient-recalled sequences are used.

Acute viral encephalitis may cause patients to present themselves with fever and obtundation (Fig. 8); initially they show no findings on MRI or CT scans. Generally, however, territorial edema predominating in the cortex and its subjacent white matter is seen. Herpes encephalitis requires rapid diagnosis and therapy and typically involves the temporal lobes and insula, sparing the medial basal ganglia. Treatment

should be based on clinical suspicion because early imaging may be negative, and delay in therapy may lead to permanent sequelae (Fig. 9). Small foci of hemorrhage and bilaterality are clues to the diagnosis.

Abscesses can be multiple in patients with systemic disease, particularly in immunocompromised hosts. Immunocompromised individuals may demonstrate target-like lesions suggesting toxoplasmosis (although the multiplicity of findings in these individuals is too broad for consideration here) (Fig. 10).

Extraaxial empyema generally is seen in the sickest of patients and is shown by contrast-en-

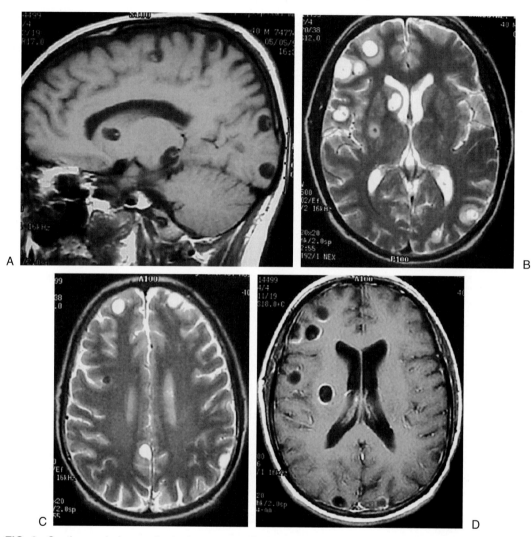

FIG. 6. Cysticercosis in a patient who presented with a seizure. **A:** T1-weighted sagittal sequence demonstrates numerous fluid-filled cysts in the brain, with central isointense nodules suggesting scolex within the cyst. **B** and **C:** T2-weighted axial sequences demonstrate the high signal intensity of the cysts, with several showing small foci of low signal intensity suggesting the calcific scolex in the fluid-filled cyst. Higher slice demonstrates a focal low signal intensity nodule in the deep white matter suggesting a calcified lesion. Calcification is the end stage of the organism's previously active status. **D:** Contrast-enhanced T1-weighted image demonstrates the ring-enhancing nature of still-living cysts. The enhancing periphery is caused by inflammation as the cyst is dying.

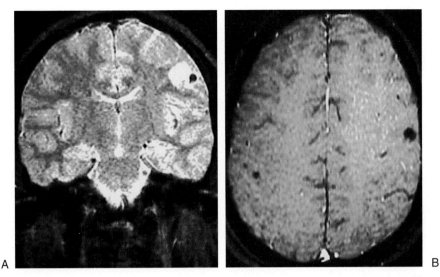

FIG. 7. Cysticercosis in a Hispanic patient with new seizure. **A:** T2-weighted coronal study demonstrates an enhancing subcortical lesion with low signal intensity. This was the only lesion seen on the routine magnetic resonance imaging study. **B:** Gradient-recalled axial slice demonstrates numerous small foci of low signal intensity consistent with calcifications from previous cysticercosis.

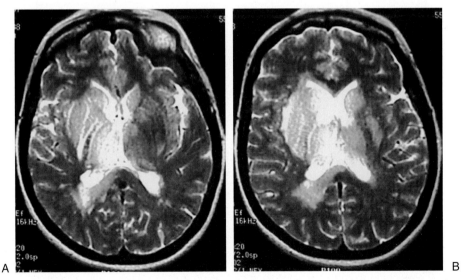

FIG. 8. Acute encephalitis/ventriculitis in a 55-year-old woman admitted for 24-hour history of stupor. Patient was obtundent on admission. Lumbar puncture revealed 580 white blood cells, with a very high protein content. **A** and **B:** T2-weighted axial sequences demonstrate diffuse edema within the basal ganglia; this extended into the white matter of the centrum semiovale on higher cuts. (*Figure continues.*)

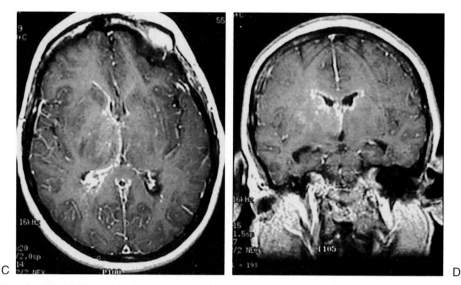

FIG. 8. *(Continued.)* **C** and **D:** Note the ependymal enhancement on the axial and coronal postcontrast T1-weighted images. Patient made steady improvement over the next 4 days, with marked improvement in lumbar puncture findings. She was discharged on the fifth hospital day.

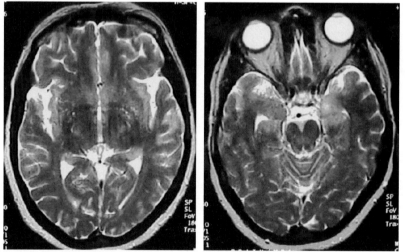

FIG. 9. Herpes encephalitis in a 60-year-old woman with acute disorientation progressing to delirium. **A** and **B:** T2-weighted axial sequences demonstrate no definite abnormality except for equivocal increased signal within the uncus of the left temporal lobe. (*Figure continues.*)

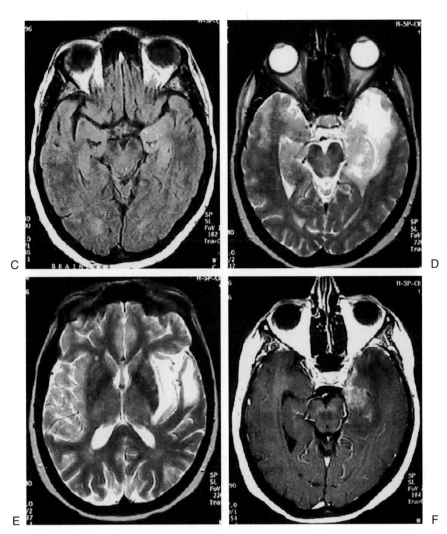

FIG. 9. *(Continued).* **C:** FLAIR sequence on the date of admission strengthens the suspicion of deep temporal abnormality. Differential diagnosis included ischemia, deep temporal astrocytoma, and herpes encephalitis. Patient was started on prophylactic acyclovir therapy. **D** and **E:** T2-weighted axial sequences obtained after 3 days demonstrate marked progression of abnormality in the left temporal lobe, consistent with the evolution of herpes encephalitis, which was subsequently proven by cerebrospinal fluid sampling. Note sparing of the basal ganglia. **F:** T1-weighted axial image after contrast injection demonstrates only mild enhancement of the diffuse abnormality in the deep temporal region.

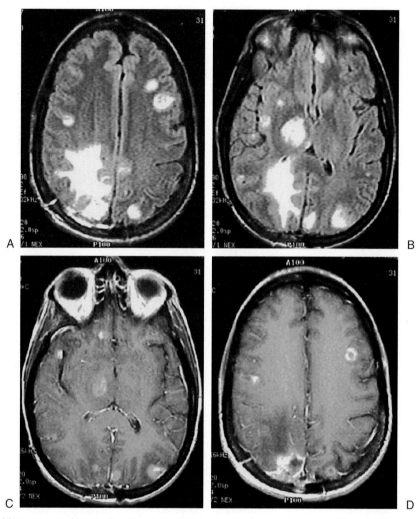

FIG. 10. Young man with acquired immunodeficiency syndrome. **A** and **B:** T2-weighted axial images demonstrate numerous ringlike lesions, some with vasogenic edema. **C** and **D:** Contrast-enhanced study verifies the enhancing nature of the lesions. Toxoplasmosis and *Staphylococcus aureus* were cultured from a biopsy specimen.

hanced sequences in particular (see Fig. 2). When seen in association with temporal infections in the child (otitis media, mastoiditis), dural sinus occlusion and venous infarction may occur as well as hydrocephalus due to the sinus occlusion. *Haemophilus influenzae* meningitis can produce sterile subdural fluid collections in the infant. Herpes encephalitis in this age group presents in a diffuse fashion (unlike the adult),

demonstrating generalized brain swelling on imaging with focal and ventricular compression, decreased density diffusely on CT, or increased signal elevation on T2-weighted images with MRI.

Ependymal and subependymal enhancement can be seen in immunocompromised hosts with cytomegalovirus infection. Small nonenhancing cysts in the basal ganglial regions shown in

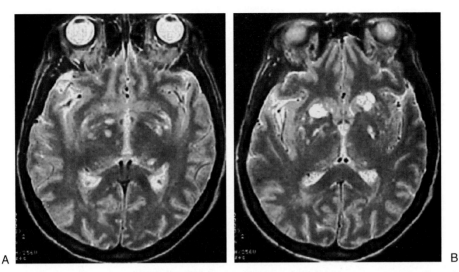

A   B

FIG. 11. Cryptococcosis in a patient with confusion and meningeal signs. **A** and **B:** T2-weighted axial sequences demonstrate small round high signal intensity foci in the low basal ganglial region. Lumbar puncture verified cryptococcosis in this nonimmunocompromised individual. T1-weighted axial sequences typically show low signal intensity within these nonenhancing foci.

these same individuals are associated with cryptococcosis (Fig. 11), the gelatinous cysts invading the expanded Virchow-Robin spaces from the basal cisterns.

V. SENSITIVITY AND SPECIFICITY

The sensitivity of MRI and especially CT to early meningitis and even early viral encephalitis is limited. The early stages of parenchymal bacterial infection are, however, readily demonstrated because of the elevated water content from the breakdown of the blood–brain barrier and resulting edema. This is particularly true with MRI. Extraaxial collections are readily depicted by the multiplanar/multiparametric capabilities of MRI.

VI. DIFFERENTIAL DIAGNOSIS

A. Metastatic Disease

Ring-enhancing lesions are common with metastases and may simulate abscesses. However, such patients rarely are as acutely ill as the in-

fected patient. Leptomeningeal enhancement of carcinomatous meningitis can be indistinguishable from infectious meningitis; thus, again clinical data and CSF sampling may be vital to make the distinction (Fig. 12).

B. Primary Brain Tumor

The gliomas can produce ring-enhancing lesions, but typically their enhancing border is garland shaped rather than circular, and the degree of edema is less given the size of the lesion (Fig. 13). Infiltrative temporal astrocytoma can simulate herpes infection but rarely is the presentation acute (seizure being the exception).

C. Infarction

Single and particularly multifocal infarcts can occasionally simulate early cerebritis as can the brain lesions of eclampsia or hypertensive encephalopathy. However, the gray matter predominates in involvement by infarction or eclampsia and the typical clinical setting of these

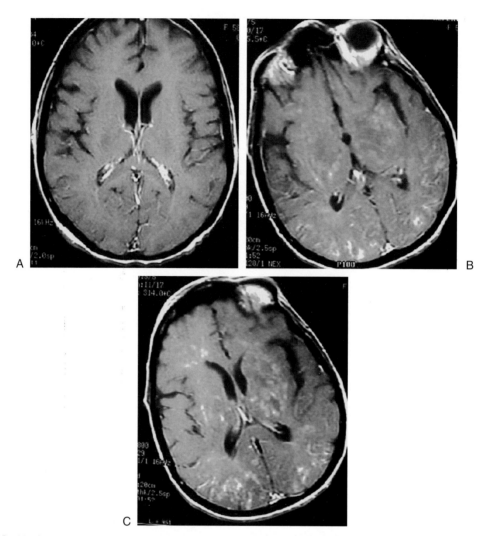

FIG. 12. Leptomeningeal metastatic disease in a 58-year-old woman with history of breast cancer. **A:** T1-weighted contrast-enhanced scan demonstrates no appreciable abnormality (done for onset of cranial neuropathy). **B** and **C:** Postcontrast T1-weighted axial images obtained 6 weeks later demonstrate diffuse leptomeningeal and Virchow-Robin space infiltration disease. Lumbar puncture verified extensive leptomeningeal carcinomatosis.

latter entities usually distinguishes them from infection.

D. Demyelinating and Other Disease

Occasionally, tumefactive multiple sclerosis and acute disseminated encephalomyelitis (ADEM) can mimic infection with bizarre garland or ring-enhancing lesions being shown after contrast injection (Fig. 14). These generally have a less symmetric shape as compared to the round capsular stage of infection, produce less edema and mass effect, and involve the deep white matter as opposed to the more peripheral gray-white matter junctional zones. ADEM and sarcoid can produce enhancement of cranial nerves, with sarcoid also causing meningeal/

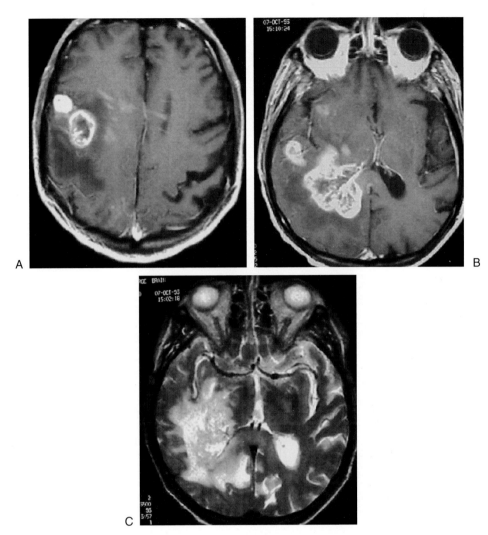

FIG. 13. High-grade multifocal astrocytoma. **A** and **B:** Some of the enhancing lesions suggest the possibility of abscess formation. However, the enhancing border is atypical for abscess. **C:** T2-weighted axial study demonstrates the dramatic lesion with relatively little mass effect and vasogenic edema given the large extent of brain involved.

cortical-enhancing patchy or nodular lesions occasionally simulating granulomatous meningitis.

VII. PITFALLS

Subarachnoid hemorrhage is a clinical mimic of meningitis, as patients will be seen with acute onset of neurologic change, severe headache, and meningism, again emphasizing the importance of lumbar puncture in cases of negative MRI or CT, which can miss subarachnoid hemorrhage in 5% to 7% of cases. Unusual vasculitic conditions associated with systemic autoimmune disorders, including systemic lupus erythematosus, can produce lesions and symptoms similar to multifocal cerebritis. Fever may be part of the presentation in these patients, as opposed to the typical primary vasculitic conditions involving the CNS. Patients on chronic steroid therapy can demonstrate remarkably advanced stages of infection despite minimal

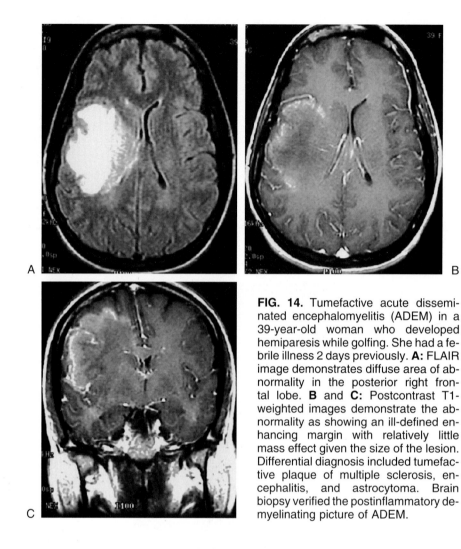

FIG. 14. Tumefactive acute disseminated encephalomyelitis (ADEM) in a 39-year-old woman who developed hemiparesis while golfing. She had a febrile illness 2 days previously. **A:** FLAIR image demonstrates diffuse area of abnormality in the posterior right frontal lobe. **B** and **C:** Postcontrast T1-weighted images demonstrate the abnormality as showing an ill-defined enhancing margin with relatively little mass effect given the size of the lesion. Differential diagnosis included tumefactive plaque of multiple sclerosis, encephalitis, and astrocytoma. Brain biopsy verified the postinflammatory demyelinating picture of ADEM.

clinical symptomatology. Certain fungi, especially aspergillosis, which invade vessels, can produce atypical lesions with features of hemorrhagic infarction masking the inflammatory pathophysiology.

VIII. SUGGESTED READINGS

Britt RH, Enzmann DR. Clinical stages of human brain abscesses on serial CT scans after contrast infusion. *J Neurosurg* 1983;59:972–989.

Gero B, Sze G, Sharif H. MR imaging of intradural inflammatory diseases of the spine. *AJNR Am J Neuroradiol* 1991;12:1009–1019.

Grafe MR, Press GA, Berthoty DP, Hesselink JR, Wiley CA. Abnormalities of the brain in AIDS patients: correlation of postmortem MR findings with neuropathology. *AJNR Am J Neuroradiol* 1990;11:905–911.

Jensen MC, Brant-Zawadzki M. MR imaging of the brain in patients with AIDS: value of routine use of IV gadopentetate dimeglumine. *AJR Am J Radiol* 1993;160:153–157.

Schroth G, Kretzschmar K, Gawehn J, Voigt K. Advantage of magnetic resonance imaging in the diagnosis of cerebral infections. *Neuroradiology* 1987;29:120–126.

4

Acute Myelopathy

Michael Brant-Zawadzki

I. CLINICAL OVERVIEW

The sudden onset of dysfunction in the spinal cord is analogous to the stroke syndrome in the brain, necessitating emergency diagnosis and treatment, when possible, to prevent permanent neurologic dysfunction. Acute myelopathy is seen less often than its brain counterpart, but it still relies on rapid diagnostic imaging for triage of patients to appropriate therapy. Although the entities in the differential diagnosis are similar to those affecting the brain, the list of insults has a different order of causes. Perhaps the most common cause of acute myelopathy syndromes necessitating imaging is compression caused by spinal metastases, the rapid diagnosis of which allows tailored radiation therapy (or occasionally surgery) and preservation or restoration of normal cord function. Traumatic insults also are common causes of acute myelopathy. Computed tomography (CT), and particularly magnetic resonance imaging (MRI), have replaced myelography in the first step of imaging patients with acute myelopathy. These patients are often difficult to position and maneuver as necessary for thorough myelography, problems overcome by the cross-sectional and three-dimensional capabilities of the modern imaging tools, which also possess rapid speed of diagnosis as a major advantage.

II. IMAGING STRATEGY

An MRI is unquestionably superior for depicting the spinal cord, surrounding subarachnoid space, and even the spinal bony architecture, being outperformed only in the latter by CT when detection of fractures is important. CT, es-

pecially with use of intrathecal nonionic contrast (CT myelography), can substitute for MRI albeit necessitating some invasiveness and limiting evaluation of the cord only to morphologic alteration as compared to the ability of MRI to characterize intrinsic cord tissue alteration. Conventional myelography is no longer needed when MRI and CT are available.

III. TECHNIQUE

Using MRI, the region of clinical interest is best studied with a matched field of view selection and use of surface (or phased array) coils. A combination technique of T1-weighted sagittal, T2-weighted spin echo sagittal, and gradient echo axial imaging is optimal for screening the cord, canal, and column morphology (T1-weighted) and intrinsic cord (and other soft tissue) characteristics (T2-weighted). The combination of techniques is also useful for detection of acute or subacute blood (gradient echo axial and T1-weighted). Sections should be thin (3 to 4 mm) and an image matrix chosen to provide 1 mm or better in-plane resolution. Pulse-gaiting can be used to diminish pulsation phase artifact from the cerebrospinal fluid (CSF). Intravenous paramagnetic contrast agents are useful to detect lesion borders within a diffuse zone of cord edema or to delineate the occasional presence of abnormal vascular structures.

When using CT, thin-section technique (1 to 1.5 mm in the cervical and 3 to 5 mm in the thoracolumbar regions) is needed. Five to 8 mL of nonionic intrathecal dye introduced into the lumbar canal (or cervical canal via C-1 to C-2 level lateral approach) provides adequate opacification of the subarachnoid space to detect intrinsic alteration of cord morphology and its extrinsic compression. Multiplanar reformations can be useful in selected instances for visualizing three-dimensional relationships.

IV. FINDINGS

In general, acute myelopathy produces deformity of the cord either on the basis of intrinsic swelling or extrinsic compression, both features being readily shown by MRI and CT myelography (Fig. 1). In certain diseases, such as multiple sclerosis, acute disseminated encephalomyelitis (ADEM), acute infarction, and even viral myelitis, small lesions that produce signal intensity increase on T2-weighted imaging or enhancement with contrast on MRI may not cause cord swelling and thus may be missed in CT myelography. Compressive lesions such as extruded discs typically efface the CSF space (Fig. 2), or if originating in the bony elements, they will demonstrate bony destruction or at least marrow infiltration (shown as decreased marrow

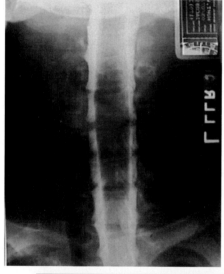

A

FIG. 1. Necrotizing amebic myelitis. Patient developed subacute left upper extremity weakness in coordination with paresthesia and neck pain and was admitted with increasing mental confusion and disorientation. **A:** Anteroposterior view of myelogram demonstrates findings suggestive of cord swelling. **B:** Postmyelography computed tomography (CT) scan verifies the increased diameter of the cord in the midcervical segment (normally, the C-5 to C-7 segment of the cervical cord is the widest). **C:** T2-weighted sagittal study of magnetic resonance imaging (MRI) shows diffuse cord swelling and edema within the C-3 to C-6 segment of the cervical cord. The subsequent course was stormy; the patient developed coma and died 5 days after admission. *Acanthoamoeba* was the offending organism for diffuse encephalomyelitis observed at autopsy. Note that noninvasive MRI study provided comparable (if not superior) information to the myelographic/CT studies.

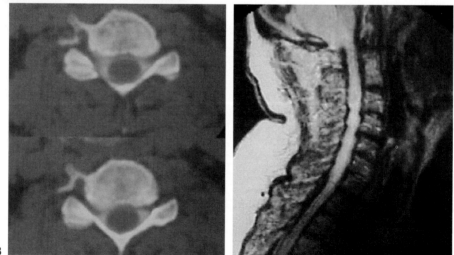

B   C

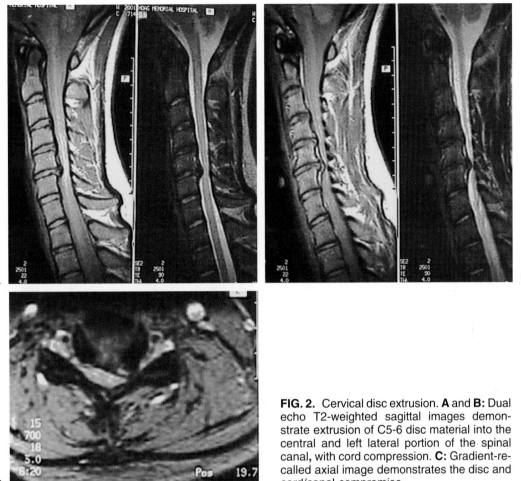

FIG. 2. Cervical disc extrusion. **A** and **B:** Dual echo T2-weighted sagittal images demonstrate extrusion of C5-6 disc material into the central and left lateral portion of the spinal canal, with cord compression. **C:** Gradient-recalled axial image demonstrates the disc and cord/canal compromise.

signal on T1-weighted imaging and increased signal on T2-weighted imaging). Hemorrhage secondary to tumor, intravenous malformation, or spontaneous epidural bleeding can produce characteristic signal intensity elevation on T1-weighted images (Fig. 3) or lowered signal intensity on gradient echo sequences. Acute hemorrhage may not show the characteristic high signal (see later).

V. SENSITIVITY AND SPECIFICITY

Magnetic resonance imaging clearly outperforms CT myelography in the detection of intrinsic cord disease causing myelopathy. Small acute demyelinating plaques (Fig. 4), ischemic insults (Fig. 5), inflammatory lesions, and even intrinsic hemorrhagic foci alter MRI signal intensity but not the shape of the cord. Specificity of the particular diagnosis is poor, necessitating correlation of imaging, clinical, and laboratory (especially CSF sampling) data. Sensitivity for detection of an extramedullary lesion compressing the cord is extremely high for both MRI and CT myelography.

VI. DIFFERENTIAL DIAGNOSIS

A. Acute Compression Fracture

Bony retropulsion compressing the cord can be caused by trauma, osteoporosis, and patho-

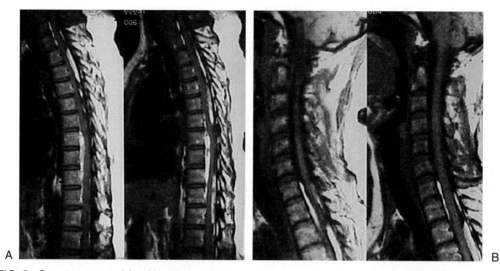

FIG. 3. Spontaneous epidural hematoma in a woman, aged 39, admitted with severe headache and cervical radiculopathy of 2 days' duration; onset followed an argument with her husband. **A** and **B:** T1-weighted sagittal sequences in the thoracic and cervical spine demonstrate lobulated epidural collections with high signal intensity typical for blood.

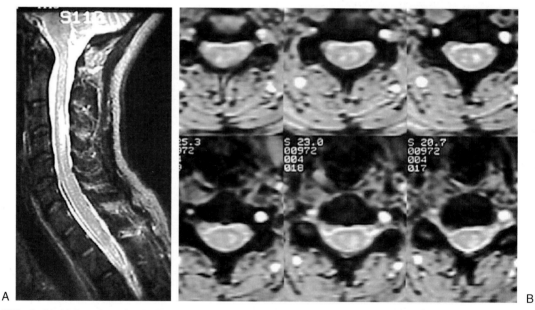

FIG. 4. Multiple sclerosis. **A:** T2-weighted sagittal sequence demonstrates the flame-shaped high signal intensity within the cervical spinal cord, predominating in the central and dorsal region. **B:** Consecutive axial gradient-recalled sequences demonstrate the coalescent demyelinating plaques in this segment.

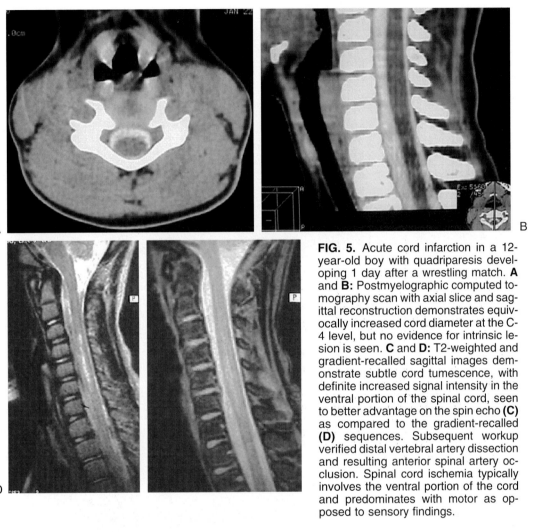

A

B

C,D

FIG. 5. Acute cord infarction in a 12-year-old boy with quadriparesis developing 1 day after a wrestling match. **A** and **B:** Postmyelographic computed tomography scan with axial slice and sagittal reconstruction demonstrates equivocally increased cord diameter at the C-4 level, but no evidence for intrinsic lesion is seen. **C** and **D:** T2-weighted and gradient-recalled sagittal images demonstrate subtle cord tumescence, with definite increased signal intensity in the ventral portion of the spinal cord, seen to better advantage on the spin echo **(C)** as compared to the gradient-recalled **(D)** sequences. Subsequent workup verified distal vertebral artery dissection and resulting anterior spinal artery occlusion. Spinal cord ischemia typically involves the ventral portion of the cord and predominates with motor as opposed to sensory findings.

logic fracture (Figs. 6 and 7). CT myelography cannot differentiate among these, except in instances when gross bony destruction indicative of either a neoplastic or infectious process is shown. In general, traumatic and osteoporotic compression fractures show preservation of some normal marrow signal on MRI, especially in the region of the pedicles. Occasionally, diffuse edema from a benign compression fracture simulates diffuse infiltration in the vertebral body; if the pedicles are involved, tumor is much more likely. Significant soft tissue mass surrounding the compressed vertebral body or in the epidural space suggests a neoplastic or infec-

tious pathology, the latter especially so if the adjacent disc interspace is destroyed and the next vertebral body is invaded.

B. Acute Myelitis

Multiple sclerosis (see Fig. 4), viral myelitis (Fig. 8), postinfectious myelitis (as part of ADEM), or nonspecific transverse myelitis can all lead to focal signal intensity increase on MRI with T2-weighted imaging. Multiple sclerosis tends to involve only one to three segments of the cord and predominates in the dorsal columns while showing minimal or no mass effect. Viral

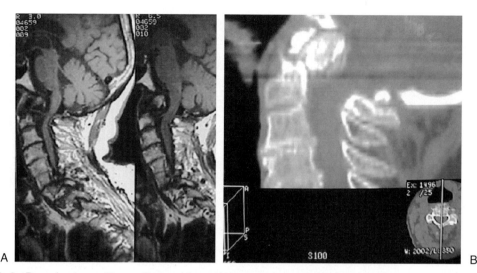

FIG. 6. Dens fracture with spastic quadriparesis in woman, aged 74. **A:** Sagittal magnetic resonance T1-weighted images demonstrate the nonunion of the dens with the parent atlas, retropulsion of the dens, and cord compression. Normal marrow signal intensity is highly suggestive of chronic nonunion as opposed to acute fracture, which would show edema of the marrow (low signal on T1-, high signal on T2-weighted images). **B:** Computed tomography (CT) scan demonstrates the same fracture, with little information regarding the degree of cord compromise. It is difficult to differentiate acute from chronic dens fracture on the CT study.

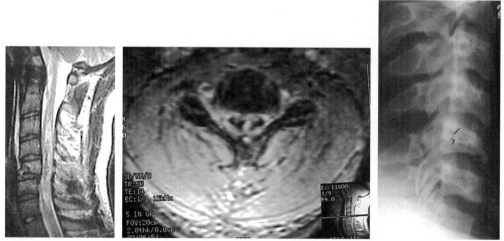

FIG. 7. Paraplegia after cervical spine trauma. **A** and **B:** T2-weighted sagittal and axial gradient-recalled sequences demonstrate cord compression and intrinsic cord alteration including low signal components consistent with magnetic susceptibility effects of hemorrhage. This heralds a grave prognosis for any recovery of cord function. **C:** Lateral plain x-ray demonstrates the acute compression fracture. Note the distracted spinous processes indicating soft tissue injury. The sagittal T2-weighted image **(A)** verifies the presence of anterior longitudinal ligament trauma by virtue of high signal intensity immediately anterior to the vertebral bodies in the mid and high cervical region.

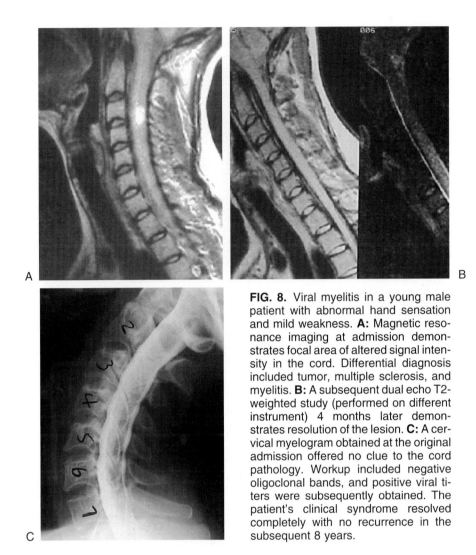

A

B

C

FIG. 8. Viral myelitis in a young male patient with abnormal hand sensation and mild weakness. **A:** Magnetic resonance imaging at admission demonstrates focal area of altered signal intensity in the cord. Differential diagnosis included tumor, multiple sclerosis, and myelitis. **B:** A subsequent dual echo T2-weighted study (performed on different instrument) 4 months later demonstrates resolution of the lesion. **C:** A cervical myelogram obtained at the original admission offered no clue to the cord pathology. Workup included negative oligoclonal bands, and positive viral titers were subsequently obtained. The patient's clinical syndrome resolved completely with no recurrence in the subsequent 8 years.

myelitis also tends to be focal but shows more mass effect early. Transverse myelitis demonstrates much more extensive segmental involvement of the cord with diffuse swelling and edema (Fig. 9). All of these entities may demonstrate enhancement after contrast injection, albeit inconstantly.

C. Vascular Insults

Cord infarction typically involves the central or ventral portion of the cord in the low thoracic region or conus and is due to occlusion of the single major vascular supply (anterior spinal artery of Adamkiewicz) (see Fig. 5). Little swelling is seen in the earliest stages of such infarcts. Clinical history of sudden loss of motor (more than sensory) function always with aortic dissection, abdominal aortic aneurysm, or accelerated atherosclerosis is helpful. This diagnosis is difficult on CT myelographic imaging alone. MRI more easily shows the hyperintensity of the lesion on T2-weighted images. Dural or arteriovenous malformations may lead to sudden venous infarcts due to stasis and thrombosis of the medullary venous drainage, although their typical presentation is of a subacute or chronic progressive paresis. Serpentine vascular channels on the

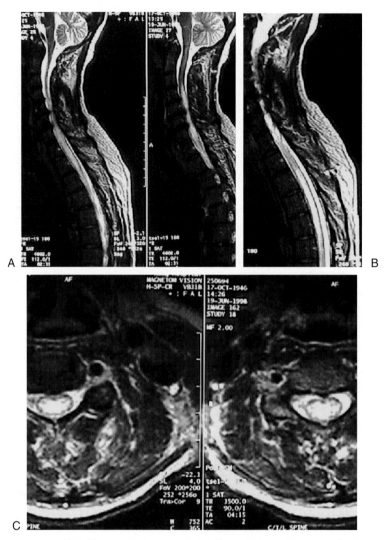

FIG. 9. Transverse myelitis. The patient presented with acute onset of paraplegia over the course of 12 hours. Cerebrospinal fluid showed high protein and 500 white blood cells. **A** and **B:** Selected T2-weighted sagittal images demonstrate diffuse edema and swelling of the cervical and thoracic cord, the lesion extending from the C-3 to the C-4 level down to the midthoracic cervical spinal cord. **C:** Transverse axial images demonstrate the edematous swollen cord as well.

dorsal surface of the cord are a helpful clue, either on MRI or CT myelography (conventional myelography with supine patient positioning may have a role when this diagnosis is suspected). If found, such lesions should be further investigated with spinal angiography.

Hemorrhage into the cord is readily depicted by MRI and suggests an underlying pathology such as arteriovenous malformation or tumor (Fig. 10). Spontaneous epidural hemorrhage is probably of venous origin and can occur with vigorous exercise or minor trauma, particularly in patients with bleeding diathesis (Figs. 11 and 12). Clinical signs are typically greater in the sensory arena as compared to the motor functions. A lumpy-bumpy epidural lesion is shown,

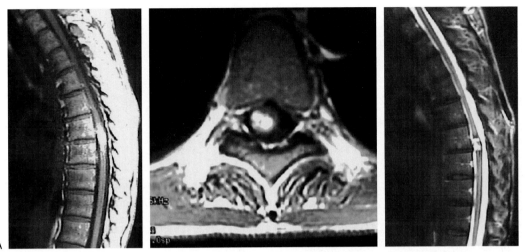

FIG. 10. Intramedullary hemorrhage. **A** and **B:** T1-weighted sagittal and axial sequences demonstrate high signal intensity within the cord substance in the midthoracic level. **C:** T2-weighted sagittal image demonstrates the high signal of the lesion, as well as peripheral low signal intensity trailing into the cord substance. An occult arteriovenous malformation was diagnosed based on lack of acute myelopathy and only mild spasticity. This lesion is analogous to occult arteriovenous malformation in the brain, which typically presents with minimal clinical signs despite the striking appearance of the lesion.

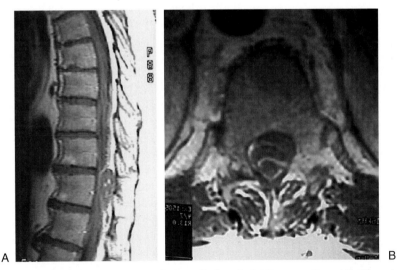

FIG. 11. Epidural hematoma in patient on Coumadin (warfarin) therapy. **A** and **B:** T1-weighted sagittal and axial (postcontrast) images demonstrate a well-circumscribed oval lesion with punctate high signal foci contained by a relatively isointense loculation, indenting the posterior spinal cord at the T-11 level. The differential diagnosis included synovial cyst and epidural empyema (see Fig. 16). The localized nature and low signal intensity of this hematoma precluded absolute characterization before surgery.

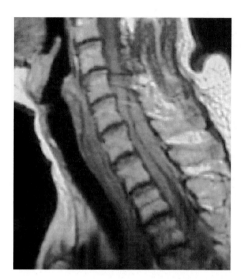

FIG. 12. Spontaneous epidural hematoma. T1-weighted sagittal image demonstrates more typical appearance of acute epidural hematoma with diffuse mass in the posterior epidural space compressing the spinal cord. This patient was taking nonsteroidal anti-inflammatory agents.

which may extend over numerous segments or be relatively localized.

D. Traumatic Myelopathy

Traumatic myelopathy is typically associated with either disc extrusion or underlying spondylosis, congenital spinal stenosis, and even ossification of the posterior longitudinal ligament (Fig. 13), when not caused by frank bony disruption and subluxation directly. Typically, the cord will demonstrate either simply compression by the abnormalities mentioned, which may be potentially reversible surgically, or intrinsic signal intensity elevation on T2-weighted images when edematous contusion is present (Fig. 14). Demonstration of lower signal intensity on gradient-recalled sequences is indicative of hemorrhage and heralds a worse prognosis (permanent neurologic deficit is more likely in such cases; see Fig. 7). Recovery of most if not all function is more likely when myelopathy after trauma is associated with decreased canal size and no signal change in the cord or only subtle signal increase or morphologic alteration.

VII. PITFALLS

Signal intensity elevation in the cord on T2-weighted imaging is frequently artifactual, especially when exaggerated spinal canal size leads to prominent CSF pulsation artifact propagated in the phase-encoding direction. Such signal intensity increase is typically curvilinear and conforms to the curve of the CSF column on sagittal images. Acute myelopathy in its earliest stages, especially that caused by ischemia or a demyelinating lesion, may show no changes. Profound motor myelopathy of Guillan-Barré syndrome may have no cord changes whatsoever but will demonstrate cauda equina enhancement (Fig. 15). Similarly, inflammatory or carcinomatous meningeal involvement is seen only after intravenous contrast injection on MRI, although increased size of the nerve roots and clumping on CT myelography or T2-weighted images can be a strong clue. Epidural collections without bony involvement causing acute myelopathy are typically hematomas (see earlier), but occasionally epidural abscess may be primarily localized in the epidural space (Fig. 16), as opposed to secondary involvement of it from discitis (Fig. 17) or vertebral osteomyelitis (Fig. 18).

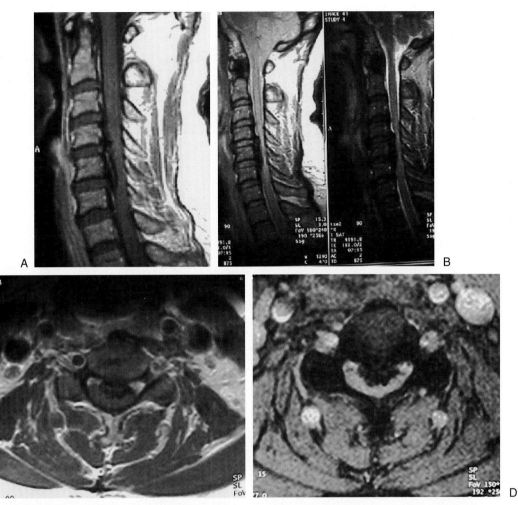

FIG. 13. Ossified posterior longitudinal ligament, paraparesis after hyperextension. **A** and **B:** T1-
and T2-weighted sagittal images demonstrate the marked spinal stenosis and cord impingement at
the C-5 level, caused by a shardlike projection from the posterior aspect of the vertebral bodies.
Note the relatively isointense signal within the center of the projection when comparing with bone
marrow signal. This is a strong clue to the entity representing ossification, given the very low signal
of cortical bone surrounding its marrow space. **C** and **D:** T1-weighted and gradient-recalled axial
sequences, respectively, demonstrate moderately severe canal compromise and cord impingement;
note the exaggeration of the lesion by the gradient echo technique caused by magnetic susceptibility
artifact. Gradient-recalled sequences can overestimate the degree of stenosis in the spine by approximately 10% to 20% because of the "blooming" at the interface of tissues with marked disparity of
magnetic susceptibility.

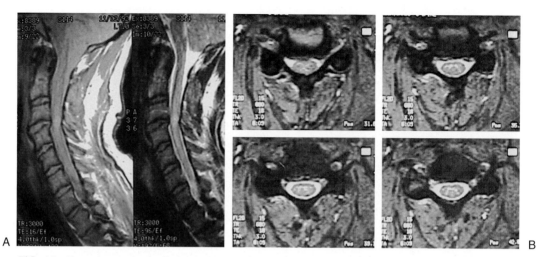

A   B

FIG. 14. Post-traumatic cord edema after diving accident; quadriparesis. **A:** Dual echo T2-weighted sagittal images demonstrate the presence of a flame-shaped high signal intensity lesion in the cord posterior to the protruding disc at the C-3 to C-4 level. Note absence of edema in the anterior longitudinal ligament. The underlying stenosis produced by the degenerated disc protrusion and the relatively small canal, combined with hyperextension, caused the cord contusion. **B:** Contiguous gradient-recalled axial sequences at the C3-4 interspace demonstrate the broad-based disc protrusion. The cord edema is not well-shown. Note the restitution of canal cross-sectional area at the mid C-4 level. Note the absence of preferentially low signal intensity change, which would herald a hemorrhagic contusion and carry a worse prognosis (compare with Fig. 7).

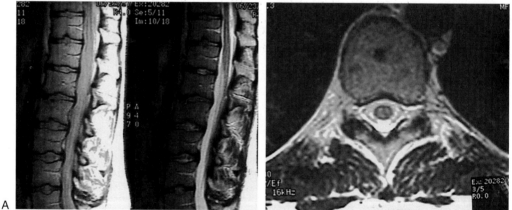

A   B

FIG. 15. Guillan-Barré syndrome. A woman, aged 39, presented with rapid onset of ascending paralysis. **A** and **B:** T2-weighted sagittal and axial sequences show no evidence of conus edema or other abnormality. *Figure continues.*

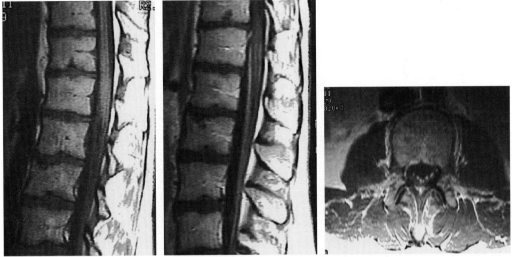

C   D,E

FIG. 15. *(Continued)* **C** and **D:** T1-weighted sagittal pre- and postcontrast sequences demonstrate prominent enhancement of the cauda equina roots on the postcontrast study. **E:** Postcontrast axial T1-weighted study verifies the discrete nerve root enhancement and slight thickening, characteristic of findings with Guillan-Barré syndrome. Differential diagnosis includes leptomeningeal seeding by tumor or leptomeningitis; however, the leptomeninges of the cord did not show the enhancement. Also, the characteristic clinical picture of predominantly motor paralysis beginning in the feet and ascending confirms the diagnosis.

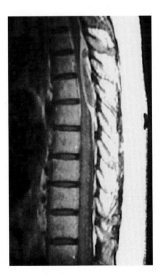

FIG. 16. Primary epidural empyema. Several-day history of pain followed by leg weakness prompted study in this woman, aged 60. T1-weighted sagittal postcontrast study demonstrates a loculated epidural collection with enhancing capsule. Pus collection was drained at surgery.

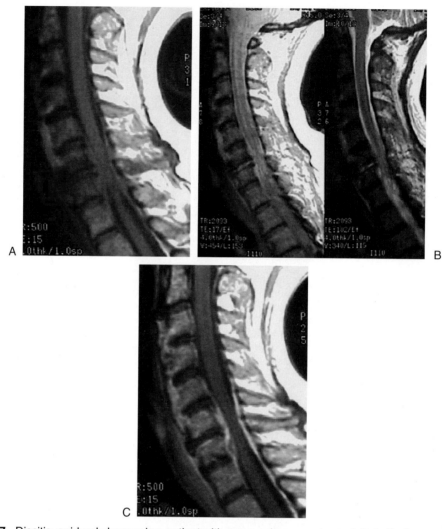

FIG. 17. Discitis, epidural abscess in a patient with arm weakness and spasticity in the lower extremities. **A:** T2-weighted sagittal study demonstrates high signal intensity within the C6-7 disc interspace, as well as a small amount of edema at the C-5 to C-6 level in the prevertebral soft tissues. **B** and **C:** T1-weighted sagittal pre- and postcontrast sequences demonstrate the low signal intensity of the vertebral bodies adjacent to the abnormal disc due to edema and the epidural soft tissue collection, which enhances predominantly after contrast injection, impinging on the cord. At surgery, granulation tissue with microabscesses was found. This is a typical appearance of early discitis and epidural abscess (which really is granulation tissue responding to the infection in the disc interspace or the vertebral body with microabscesses within the granulation tissue). The one atypical feature here is lack of enhancement within the abnormal disc interspace itself. The vertebral bodies do enhance when comparing the pre- and postcontrast images.

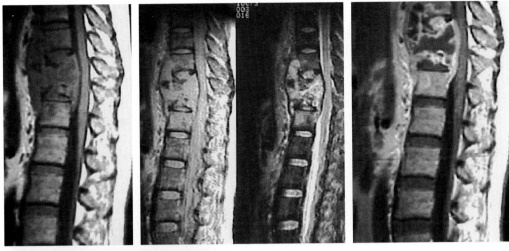

A

B,C

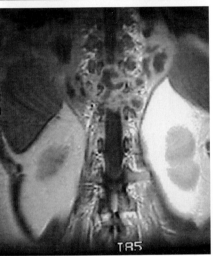

D

FIG. 18. Tubercular vertebral osteomyelitis (Pott's disease). **A** and **B:** T1-weighted and T2-weighted sagittal dual echo sequences demonstrate the destructive lesions of the vertebral bodies at the T-10 to T-11 level. Note some sparing of the interspace between the vertebral bodies and the epidural as well as prevertebral mass. **C:** Postcontrast T1-weighted sagittal study demonstrates enhancement of the periphery of the loculated masses. **D:** Coronal T1-weighted image demonstrates the associated paravertebral abscesses.

VIII. SUGGESTED READINGS

An HS, Andreshak TG, Nguyen C, Williams A, Daniels D. Can we distinguish between benign versus malignant compression fractures of the spine by magnetic resonance imaging? *Spine* 1995;20:1776–1782.

Flanders AE, Schaefer DM, Doan HT, Mishkin MM, Gonzalez CF, Northrup BE. Acute cervical spine trauma: correlation of MR imaging findings with degree of neurologic deficit. *Radiology* 1990;177:25–33.

Holtas S, Heiling M, Lonntoft M. Spontaneous spinal epidural hematoma: findings at MR imaging and clinical correlation. *Radiology* 1996;199:409–413.

Mawad ME, Rivera V, Crawford S, Ramirez A, Breitbach W. Spinal cord ischemia after resection of thoracoabdominal aortic aneurysms: MR findings in 24 patients. *AJNR Am J Neuroradiol* 1990;11:987–991.

Tartaglino LM, Croul SE, Flanders AE, et al. Idiopathic acute transverse myelitis: MR imaging findings. *Radiology* 1996;201:661–669.

Tartaglino LM, Friedman DP, Flanders AE, Lublin FD, Knobler RL, Liem M. Multiple sclerosis in the spinal cord: MR appearance and correlation with clinical parameters. *Radiology* 1995;195:725–732.

5

Chest Trauma

Ann N. Leung

I. CLINICAL OVERVIEW

Injury to the chest directly causes or significantly contributes to patient death in approximately one-half of trauma-related deaths. Chest trauma is traditionally classified as penetrating or blunt depending on whether a communication between internal organs and the outside environment has been created. Penetrating injury is typically caused by missiles (gun-related injury) or knife wounds. Tissue damage in penetrating trauma is largely confined to structures directly in the path taken by the projectile with the resulting severity of injury dependent on the specific structures injured.

Blunt chest trauma accounts for the majority of chest injuries that occur in civilian populations and most commonly results from motor vehicle accidents (MVAs) and falls. Blunt chest injuries are associated with a higher mortality rate than penetrating trauma because of the higher incidence of multiple organ involvement. Direct impact produces injuries primarily to the chest wall; more important damage to intrathoracic contents results from indirect forces such as compression and decompression, differential deceleration, and shearing and torsion.

Blunt aortic injury (BAI) is the second most common cause of death after head injury in trauma-related deaths and occurs most commonly as a result of MVAs (1). In excess of 80% of affected patients die before arrival at a treatment facility. In survivors, delays in diagnosis result in higher mortality; unoperated mortality of BAI is estimated at 1% per hour for the first 48 hours after hospital admission. The anatomic sites of aortic injury are proximal descending in 93%, arch in 4%, ascending in 3%, and diaphragmatic in 1% (1). A predilection for these specific sites of involvement is dictated by the mechanism of injury. With rapid deceleration of the thorax and compression of the diaphragm, the aorta is subjected to extreme torque and compression at anatomic points of attachment (isthmus, sinuses of Valsalva, and diaphragm) where severe wall stress ultimately results in rupture. Traumatic laceration resulting from "pinching" of the aorta between the spine and anterior bony structures such as the manubrium, clavicle, and first rib has also been postulated as a potential mechanism that could explain involvement of atypical sites such as the aortic arch and proximal arch vessels.

Hemothorax is commonly seen in association with both penetrating and blunt chest trauma. Bleeding usually arises from injury of low-pressure pulmonary vessels and either subsides spontaneously or responds to treatment with simple tube thoracostomy. Approximately 10% of patients with traumatic hemothorax eventually require thoracotomy because of massive initial hemothorax or sustained bleeding into the pleural space, usually resulting from disruption of systemic thoracic veins or arteries or central pulmonary vessels.

Pneumothorax is a common finding associated with chest trauma and usually indicates the presence of a parenchymal tear that extends across visceral pleura. Tension pneumothorax develops when communication between the lung and pleural space functions as a check valve such that air enters but cannot exit the pleural space. When intrapleural pressure exceeds atmospheric pressure, venous return to the thorax is impeded and, in association with compression of the ipsilateral lung, results in severe and progressive shunting and hypoxemia.

Pulmonary contusions are defined as injuries to lung parenchyma resulting in edema and hemorrhage into interstitial and alveolar tissues. Extensive involvement, particularly when found in combination with overhydration, may result in respiratory failure.

Flail chest typically results from a direct impact and is diagnosed when three or more adjacent ribs, each fractured in two or more locations, produce a segment of chest wall that is unsupported and moves paradoxically during ventilation. This condition is important to recognize because significant ventilatory disturbances frequently develop in affected patients and arise secondary to both inefficient mechanics of chest wall motion as well as physiologic abnormalities caused by underlying pulmonary contusion.

Sternal fracture most commonly results from MVAs. Although traditionally associated with myocardial contusion and great vessel injury, the mandatory use of seat belt restraints, which has decreased the occurrence of direct precordial impact against steering wheels and ejection of car occupants, has changed the pathophysiology and diagnostic significance of sternal fractures. Several studies have demonstrated that restrained car occupants with isolated sternal fractures are not predisposed to other more serious, occult injuries.

Fractures of the thoracic spine are less common than fractures involving the cervical and lumbar regions and typically occur in flexion and axial loading. The majority of thoracic spine fractures occur in the lower thoracic region; because of the relatively large size of the spinal cord in relation to the size of the spinal canal in this region, one-half of patients with thoracic fractures have accompanying neurologic findings. Thoracic spinal injuries can be classified into four categories: compression fractures, burst fractures, seat belt-type injuries (including Chance fracture), and fracture dislocations.

Tracheobronchial disruption is a rare complication of blunt chest trauma, occurring in fewer than 1% of cases; this injury more commonly occurs in association with iatrogenic penetrating trauma. Tracheobronchial rupture associated with blunt trauma typically occurs within 2.5 cm of the carina. The most common clinical signs are dyspnea and subcutaneous emphysema present in 75% of the patients.

Traumatic esophageal perforation most commonly occurs as an iatrogenic complication after diagnostic or therapeutic procedures. The esophagus is infrequently injured by external penetrating trauma such as missile or knife wounds; however, because delays in diagnosis result in increased mortality, esophageal perforation should always be suspected when penetration involves the neck or mediastinum. Because of its more vulnerable location, the cervical esophagus is more frequently injured than is the thoracic esophagus and is involved in approximately 5% of neck wounds. Esophageal rupture after blunt chest trauma is rare and usually involves the lower third of the esophagus.

Acute diaphragmatic rupture occurs in 1% to 7% of patients after major blunt trauma. Rupture usually occurs in the weakest portion along the posterolateral aspect of the hemidiaphragm and is seen with a marked left-sided predominance attributed to the right-sided protective effects of the liver.

II. IMAGING STRATEGY

Imaging studies should be obtained only after vital signs have been stabilized. Life-threatening conditions such as cardiac tamponade, massive hemothorax, and tension pneumothorax are usually diagnosed on the basis of clinical findings and treated emergently before radiologic evaluation.

Chest radiography should be the initial imaging technique in all patients. Further evaluation using other imaging modalities may be indicated on the basis of abnormal radiographic findings or a high clinical suspicion of significant intrathoracic injury because of a causally linked mechanism of injury. In penetrating chest trauma caused by firearms, computed tomography (CT) is used to define the intracorporeal missile path with specific identification of the traversed and damaged organs and body compartments (Fig. 1).

Helical CT and transesophageal echocardiography (TEE) are cost-effective methods to evaluate hemodynamically stable patients with suspected BAI. Helical CT is often used as the imaging modality of choice in emergent situations because of its availability, speed, and ability to assess simultaneously for coexistent intrathoracic injuries. The main advantage of TEE is that it can be performed rapidly at the bedside while stabilization measures continue. Disadvantages of TEE, which have prevented its widespread use, are limited availability of skilled operators in emergent settings and lack of visualization of a 3- to 5-cm portion of the upper ascending aorta and arch branch vessels. Aortography, which remains the imaging gold standard, is reserved for situations in which helical CT or TEE evaluation is not available or is nondiagnostic.

Suspected injuries to the tracheobronchial tree and esophagus are best assessed with bronchoscopy and esophagography, respectively. A barium esophagram should always follow a water-soluble contrast examination if extravasation is not initially identified.

III. TECHNIQUE

Portable chest radiographs should be obtained with the patient in an erect position whenever possible to minimize the number of false-positive studies for BAI caused by mediastinal vascular engorgement in supine patients (Fig. 2). Radiographic evaluation of injury to the thoracic spine requires dedicated anteroposterior (AP) and lateral views centered and collimated on the thoracic spine because up to 50% of fractures may be missed on AP chest radiographs alone.

Optimized helical CT evaluation of suspected BAI consists of thin-collimation (3-mm) volumetric study acquired using high injection rates of nonionic contrast (4 to 5 mL/s of 300 mg iodine/mL) and reconstructed with overlapping increments (2 mm). CT evaluation should extend from 2 cm above the aortic arch to the diaphragm; a pitch of 2 is used to maximize z-axis coverage. Scan acquisition timed to the optimal phase of arterial opacification is achieved by performance of an initial test bolus of 10 mL of contrast; scanning delay is set to earliest time of peak contrast opacification in the thoracic aorta as measured on a generated time-density curve and typically ranges from 15 to 20 seconds. Includ-

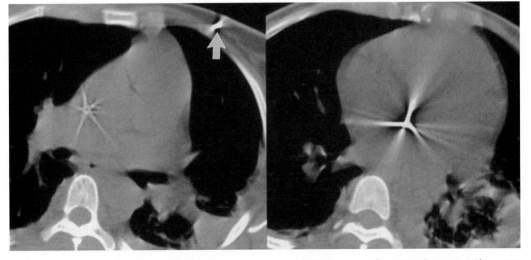

FIG. 1. Shotgun injury involving the heart in a 32-year-old woman. Computed tomography scan obtained with 3-mm collimation shows metallic pellets lodged in the left anterior chest wall (*arrow*), adjacent to the right atrium, and between the right and left atria.

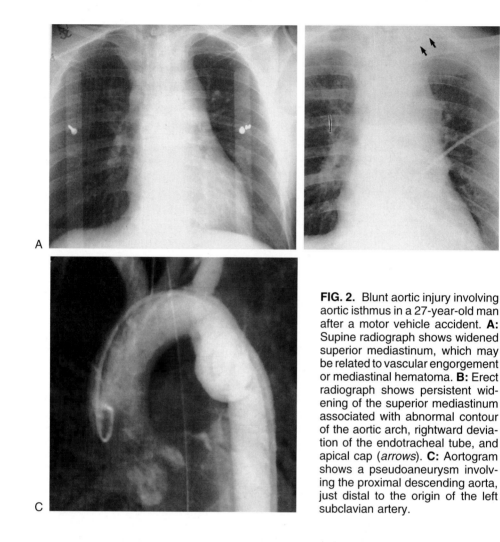

FIG. 2. Blunt aortic injury involving aortic isthmus in a 27-year-old man after a motor vehicle accident. **A:** Supine radiograph shows widened superior mediastinum, which may be related to vascular engorgement or mediastinal hematoma. **B:** Erect radiograph shows persistent widening of the superior mediastinum associated with abnormal contour of the aortic arch, rightward deviation of the endotracheal tube, and apical cap (*arrows*). **C:** Aortogram shows a pseudoaneurysm involving the proximal descending aorta, just distal to the origin of the left subclavian artery.

ing the timing bolus, the total volume of contrast administered is 130 to 140 mL.

IV. FINDINGS

All radiographic signs described in association with aortic injury represent manifestations of mediastinal hemorrhage with hematoma formation and mass effect. The most discriminating signs are loss of the aortopulmonary window, abnormal contour of the aortic arch, rightward tracheal deviation at the level of T-4, and widening of the left paraspinal line without associated vertebral fracture (Fig. 3). Other described signs of lesser discriminant value include widening of the mediastinum (subjective or more than 8 cm at the level of the aortic arch), displacement of nasogastric tube to the right at the level of T-4, and depression of the left mainstem bronchus and left apical pleural cap.

Although conventional CT scanners have only allowed reliable detection of mediastinal hematoma, an indirect and nonspecific sign of both arterial and venous vascular injury, the advent of helical scanners permits direct visualization of the site and location of aortic disruption. Incomplete lacerations of the aortic wall manifest as

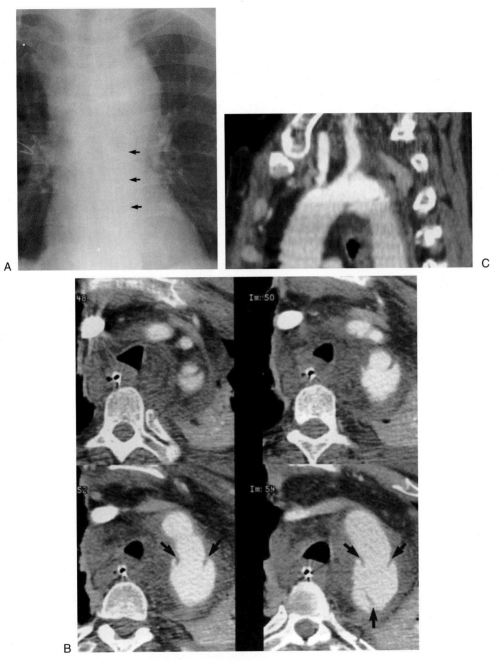

FIG. 3. Blunt aortic injury involving the aortic isthmus in a 57-year-old man after a motor vehicle accident. **A:** Supine radiograph shows widened superior mediastinum with abnormal contour of the aortic arch, rightward tracheal deviation, depression of the left mainstem bronchus, and displaced left paraspinal line (*arrows*). **B:** Spiral computed tomographic angiogram obtained with 3-mm collimation shows intimal flaps (*arrows*) involving the proximal descending aorta with pseudoaneurysm formation. **C:** Curved planar reformation shows an abnormal contour of the aortic isthmus.

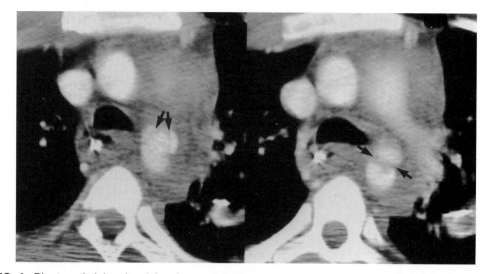

FIG. 4. Blunt aortic injury involving the aortic isthmus in a 17-year-old boy struck by train. Spiral CT scan obtained with 7-mm collimation shows intimal flaps (*arrows*) with pseudoaneurysm formation in the proximal descending aorta associated with extensive mediastinal hematoma.

areas of low attenuation, characteristically linear in appearance, that project into the opacified aortic lumen; adjacent contrast collections that extend beyond the expected aortic lumen represent pseudoaneurysms, which are contained by the aortic adventitial layer (Figs. 3 and 4).

A pneumothorax is diagnosed on chest radiographs by identification of an internally displaced visceral pleural line separated from the chest wall. Tension pneumothorax is a clinical diagnosis but may be suggested when radiographs demonstrate a pneumothorax associated with significant mass effect causing mediastinal shift and flattening or eversion of the ipsilateral hemidiaphragm (Fig. 5).

The radiographic findings of pulmonary contusion consist of consolidation in a nonsegmental distribution usually conforming to the side of trauma although involvement of the contralateral lung may also occur. Contusions become radiographically apparent within a few hours after trauma and typically show improvement within 3 days. On CT, most patients with radiographic evidence of lung contusion as a consequence of blunt chest trauma have parenchymal lacerations (2). Four distinct types of lacerations have been described and are differentiated on the basis of their CT appearance and presumed

pattern of injury. The four types with associated mechanisms of injury in decreasing order of frequency are:

- Intraparenchymal cavity sometimes containing an air–fluid level resulting from lung rup-

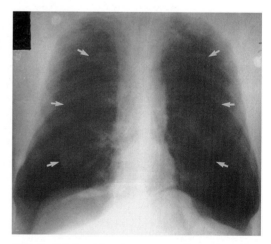

FIG. 5. Bilateral tension pneumothorax in an 80-year-old man after cardiopulmonary resuscitation. Supine radiograph shows large air collections in each pleural cavity separating visceral (*arrows*) from parietal pleura and associated with a relatively small heart size and depression of hemidiaphragms.

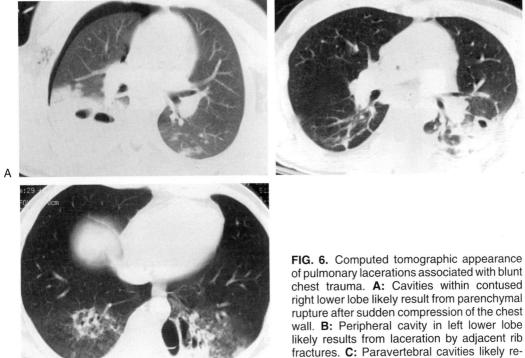

A

B

C

FIG. 6. Computed tomographic appearance of pulmonary lacerations associated with blunt chest trauma. **A:** Cavities within contused right lower lobe likely result from parenchymal rupture after sudden compression of the chest wall. **B:** Peripheral cavity in left lower lobe likely results from laceration by adjacent rib fractures. **C:** Paravertebral cavities likely result from shear of left lower lobe against vertebra.

ture following sudden chest wall compression (Fig. 6A)

- Small peripheral cavity caused by laceration from an adjacent rib fracture (Fig. 6B)
- Paravertebral cavity created by shear of lower lobe against vertebra (Fig. 6C)
- Parenchymal tear caused by pleural adhesions with sudden movement of overlying chest wall (2).

In comparison to blunt trauma, the CT appearance of a parenchymal laceration created by penetrating injury such as a gunshot or knife wound (Fig. 7) tends to have a more cylindrical shape that usually extends to the peripheral entrance site of the projectile.

Radiographic findings of tracheobronchial rupture consist of pneumomediastinum, pneumothorax refractory to chest tube drainage, and subcutaneous emphysema. Rarely, a detached lobe may be seen collapsed toward the lateral chest wall (fallen lung sign). Persistent failure of a lobe to expand after chest tube placement

in the clinical context of severe blunt trauma should suggest either bronchial rupture (Fig. 8) or foreign body obstruction (Fig. 9).

Radiographic findings associated with esophageal disruption consist of subcutaneous cervi-

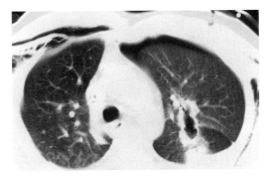

FIG. 7. Stab wound in a 34-year-old man. Computed tomography scan obtained with 7-mm collimation shows cylindrical appearance of left upper lobe parenchymal laceration with peripheral extension to wound entrance site.

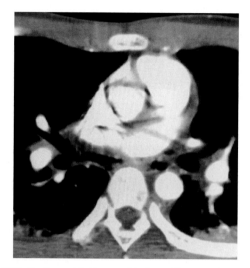

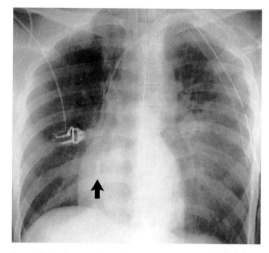

FIG. 8. Bronchial laceration in a 17-year-old boy after 45-foot fall. Computed tomography scan obtained with 3-mm collimation shows linear air tract extending from the medial wall of the bronchus intermedius into the adjacent mediastinum.

FIG. 9. Obstructive atelectasis caused by aspirated foreign body in a 19-year-old man with maxillofacial injury after a motor vehicle accident. Supine radiograph shows incisor (*arrow*) impacted in the bronchus with resulting atelectasis of the right lower lobe.

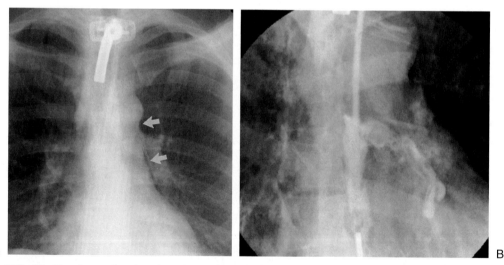

A   B

FIG. 10. Esophageal perforation after attempted dilatation of lye-induced esophageal stricture in a 28-year-old man. **A:** Posteroanterior chest radiograph shows subtle mediastinal emphysema (*arrows*). **B:** Esophagram using water-soluble contrast injected via a feeding tube shows simultaneous opacification of the esophagus and left mainstem bronchus consistent with bronchoesophageal fistula.

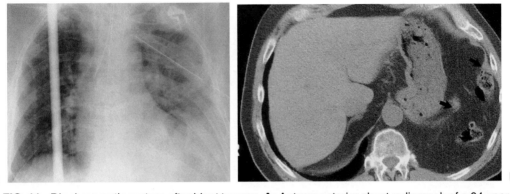

A   B

FIG. 11. Diaphragmatic rupture after blunt trauma. **A:** Anteroposterior chest radiograph of a 64-year-old man shows intrathoracic herniation of the stomach associated with multiple left-sided rib fractures and contusion of the left lung. The tip of the endotracheal tube is in the right mainstem bronchus. **B:** Computed tomography scan obtained with 7-mm collimation of a 60-year-old man shows discontinuity (*arrows*) of the left hemidiaphragm with intrathoracic herniation of the splenic flexure and mesenteric fat.

cal emphysema in cases of penetrating trauma and pneumomediastinum (Fig. 10A) and pneumothorax. Findings are similar to those associated with tracheobronchial injury but are usually less extensive. On esophagography, diagnosis of esophageal disruption is made on the basis of extraluminal extravasation of contrast (Fig. 10B).

Although the majority of patients with acute diaphragmatic rupture have abnormal chest radiographs, only a minority will have findings suggestive of the diagnosis. Findings include an aberrant course of an intragastric nasogastric tube superior to the expected location of the left hemidiaphragm and gas-containing stomach or bowel within the left hemithorax (Fig. 11A). On CT, diagnosis is made on the basis of identification of diaphragmatic discontinuity with intrathoracic herniation of abdominal contents (Fig. 11B).

V. SENSITIVITY AND SPECIFICITY

Helical CT, TEE, and aortography are all excellent methods to evaluate for BAI with reported sensitivity and specificity of 100% and 92%, 97% to 100% and 75% to 98%, and 94% and 96%, respectively (1,3–5).

VI. DIFFERENTIAL DIAGNOSIS

Mediastinal hematoma resulting in radiographic widening of the mediastinum may result from vascular (venous and arterial) or bony injury. Fractures of the sternum and spine are often accompanied by anterior mediastinal (Fig. 12) and paravertebral hematoma (Fig. 13A), respectively, which may be mistakenly attributed to great vessel injury. Although hematoma associated with these fractures usually does not cause mass effect within the middle mediastinum, CT scan may be used in problematic cases to determine the exact site of injury (see Figs. 12C and 13B).

VII. PITFALLS

Normal radiographs can occur in association with aortic injury with false-negative results reported in up to 7% of cases (1). In clinical situations in which a high index of suspicion for aortic injury exists because of either a causally linked mechanism of injury or physical evidence of severe blunt trauma, early additional imaging studies are required to exclude this potentially fatal entity.

Diagnosis of diaphragmatic rupture is missed in 50% of patients on initial presentation, likely

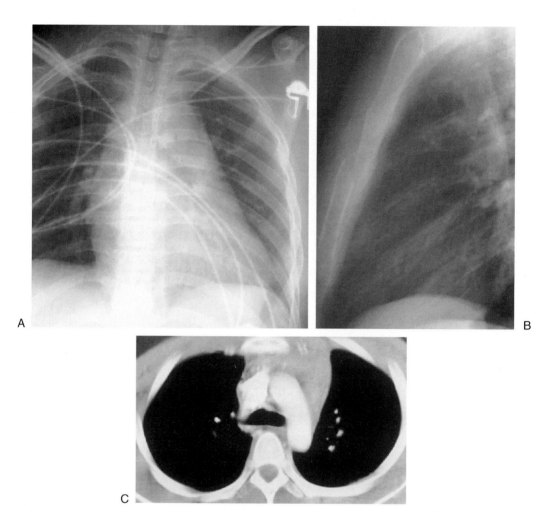

FIG. 12. Sternal fracture in an 18-year-old restrained passenger in a motor vehicle accident. **A:** Supine radiograph shows a widened superior mediastinum with an abnormal contour of aortic arch. **B:** Lateral radiograph shows displaced sternal fracture. **C:** Spiral computed tomography (CT) scan obtained with 10-mm collimation shows anterior mediastinal hematoma resulting from sternal fracture; both CT and subsequent aortogram were negative for blunt aortic injury.

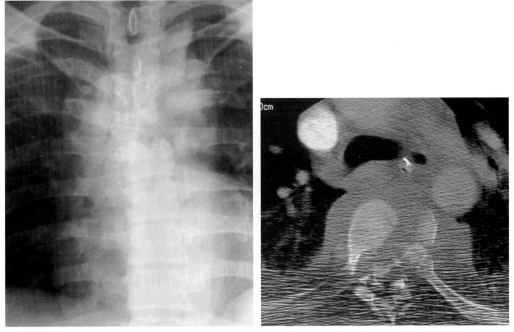

A   B

FIG. 13. Burst fracture in a 44-year-old man after a bicycle accident. **A:** Supine radiograph shows widening of the superior mediastinum with displacement of the left paraspinal line and malalignment at the T-5 to T-6 level. **B:** Computed tomography scan obtained with 10-mm collimation shows T-5 burst fracture with retropulsion of fragments into the spinal canal and associated paraspinal hematoma.

because of both a frequent association with more emergent life-threatening injuries as well as the nonspecificity of its clinical and radiographic findings. In the undetected state, the negative pressure gradient that normally exists between the pleural and peritoneal cavities can cause progressive enlargement of the diaphragmatic laceration and continued herniation of intraabdominal contents into the thorax. Late complications such as intestinal obstruction and gangrene and cardiorespiratory compromise secondary to compression occur weeks to years following injury.

VIII. REFERENCES

1. Fabian TC, Richardson D, Croce MA, et al. Prospective study of blunt aortic injury: multicenter trial of the American Association for the Surgery of Trauma. *J Trauma* 1997;42:374–383.
2. Wagner RB, Crawford WO Jr, Schimpf PP. Classification of parenchymal injuries of the lung. *Radiology* 1988;167: 77–82.
3. Mattox KL. Red River anthology. *J Trauma* 1997;42: 353–368.
4. Smith MD, Cassidy JM, Souther S, et al. Transesophageal echocardiography in the diagnosis of traumatic rupture of the aorta. *N Engl J Med* 1995;332:356–362.
5. Gavant ML, Menke PG, Fabian T, Flick PA, Graney MJ, Gold RE. Blunt traumatic aortic rupture: detection with helical CT of the chest. *Radiology* 1995;197:125–133.

6

Acute Chest Pain of Noncardiac Origin

Ann N. Leung

I. CLINICAL OVERVIEW

Chest pain is one of the most common and difficult presenting complaints that requires evaluation in the emergent setting. Because of the visceral origin of many types of chest pain, the pain often has a vague presentation with indistinct anatomic boundaries. Rapid and accurate assessment is important because chest pain may indicate the presence of potentially life-threatening conditions.

The quality and location of chest pain associated with thoracic aortic diseases are often indistinguishable; pain typically is acute in onset and involves the anterior part of the chest, the neck, or the area between the shoulders. Aortic dissection is the most common fatal condition that involves the aorta and is associated with a mortality rate as high as 1% per hour during the first 48 hours after onset of symptoms, if untreated (1). Dissection results when blood separates the layer of the aortic media, usually through a tear in the intima, which occurs most commonly in the ascending aorta adjacent to the aortic root. Peak incidence is in the sixth and seventh decades of life and common predisposing conditions include hypertension, bicuspid aortic valve, and Marfan syndrome. In young patients presenting with acute chest pain, cocaine use is an important predisposing factor that can result in aortic dissection or rupture. The Stanford classification divides dissection into those that involve the ascending aorta (type A) and require immediate surgical treatment as opposed to others that begin distal to the left subclavian artery (type B) and are amenable to medical therapy. Intramural hematoma is believed to arise from either spontaneous rupture of an atherosclerotic plaque or vasa vasorum of the aorta leading to subintimal bleeding. Essentially for purposes of management, it may be viewed as an aortic dissection without a demonstrable intimal tear; intramural hematoma involving the ascending aorta requires surgical management, whereas those beginning distal to the left subclavian artery are treated with medical therapy.

A penetrating ulcer results from ulceration of an atherosclerotic plaque that penetrates into the internal elastic lamina and allows hematoma formation within the media of the aortic wall. A penetrating ulcer typically appears as a focal ulcer with adjacent subintimal hematoma in the middle or distal third of the descending thoracic aorta; it rarely occurs in the ascending aorta or arch due to the relative sparing of these areas by atherosclerosis.

Aortic rupture and pseudoaneurysm formation are the end-stage, catastrophic complications of aortic aneurysm and any of the other potentially lethal aortic diseases previously discussed. In addition to chest pain, patients with active bleeding will also exhibit signs of hemodynamic instability on clinical examination.

Pleuritic pain, caused by irritation of parietal pleura, is characterized by aggravation with inspiration, coughing, and sneezing. A parietal pleura that lines the interior of the rib cage and outer portion of each hemidiaphragm is innervated by the neighboring intercostal nerves; referred pain is localized to the cutaneous distribution of the involved nerve over the chest wall. A parietal pleura that lines the central portion of each hemidiaphragm is innervated by the phrenic nerve; referred pain is localized to the ipsilateral shoulder or neck. Infections are the most common cause of pleuritic pain and are usually associated with dyspnea and fever. Pleural empyema refers to the presence of pus or infected fluid within the pleural space. Pneumothorax and pulmonary embolism are two conditions associated with acute pleuritic chest pain that may potentially be fatal if untreated. Dyspnea is the most common and prominent symptom in patients with pulmonary embolism (see Chapter 7); pleuritic chest pain may be associated in up to two-thirds of patients.

A persistent and unrelenting quality differentiates chest wall pain from pleuropulmonary causes of chest pain. Pancoast tumor refers to superior sulcal carcinomas, typically squamous cell in origin, that arise in the extreme apex of the lung and typically invade adjacent ribs and vertebrae, C-8 to T-2 nerve roots, sympathetic chain, and stellate ganglion. Patients complain of deep, unrelenting pain that begins in the shoulder and scapular regions and progresses to involve the arm and forearm; Horner's syndrome (ptosis, miosis, anhidrosis, and enophthalmos) is associated with stellate ganglion invasion. Simple rib fractures are a common but relatively unimportant cause of chest wall pain. Uncommonly, chest wall pain may be caused by direct extension of pulmonary infections to involve chest wall structures.

Pain arising from the esophagus is usually referred to midline structures such as the throat, neck, and sternal regions but may also involve the arms. The pain associated with esophageal perforation is typically sharp and sudden in onset and may be aggravated by swallowing and breathing. Etiologically, esophageal perforations are divided into iatrogenic and noniatrogenic types; iatrogenic perforations are more common and usually result from esophageal dilatation and, less frequently, diagnostic flexible fiberoptic esophagoscopy. Boerhaave's syndrome refers to barogenic rupture of the esophagus associated with raised intraesophageal pressure typically caused by vomiting but also reported in association with weight lifting, severe asthma, and parturition. The site of rupture in descending order of frequency is the left posterolateral aspect of the distal esophagus, the midesophagus, and the right, distal esophagus.

II. IMAGING STRATEGY

Posteroanterior and lateral chest radiographs should be the initial imaging study in evaluating patients with acute chest pain. Computed tomography (CT), multiplanar transesophageal echocardiography (TEE), and magnetic resonance imaging (MRI) are all excellent imaging techniques for evaluation of the thoracic aorta. Helical CT is often used as the imaging modality of choice in emergent situations because of its availability, speed, and ability to detect aortic dissection extension into supraaortic vessels and the abdominal aorta as well as the presence of blood in pleural and pericardial spaces. The major disadvantage of CT is that it requires the use of intravenous contrast, which may be contraindicated in patients with a history of anaphylactic reaction or renal insufficiency.

Multiplanar TEE is the modality of choice for evaluation of the thoracic aorta in hemodynamically unstable patients because it can be performed rapidly at the bedside while stabilization measures continue. The main limitations of multiplanar TEE are the strong dependence on the operator's experience, suboptimal visualization of a short segment of the ascending aorta and arch vessels, and inability to visualize distal extension of aortic dissection beyond the celiac trunk. Similar to TEE, MRI can evaluate for the presence of aortic valve regurgitation as well as provide similar anatomic characterization of the thoracic aorta as obtained with helical CT. Use of MRI is limited to hemodynamically stable patients because of limited patient access and impaired monitoring of vital signs during the examination. Cardiac pacemakers, ferromagnetic aneurysm or hemostatic clips, and ocular or otologic implants are contraindications to MRI.

Esophagography performed initially with a water-soluble contrast medium and followed by barium, if necessary, should be performed in all patients suspected of having esophageal rupture.

III. TECHNIQUE

An optimized protocol for helical CT angiogram of the thoracic aorta is described in the technique section of Chapter 5.

MRI protocols for evaluating thoracic aortic disease usually include electrocardiographic (ECG)-gated T1-weighted spin echo sequences in coronal and axial planes and three-dimensional gadolinium-enhanced magnetic resonance angiography. Cine MRI using either gradient-recalled echo or phase-contrast pulse sequences may also be performed to allow dynamic or functional assessment of aortic blood flow.

IV. FINDINGS

The most common radiographic findings associated with aortic dissection are widening of the mediastinum, widening of the aortic knob, change in configuration of the aorta between successive examinations, and displacement of calcified plaque by 10 mm or more (Fig. 1). Diagnosis of aortic dissection on any of the cross-sectional imaging modalities rests on identification of two or more luminal channels separated by an intimal flap (Fig. 2).

Intramural hematoma is diagnosed on identification of crescentic mural thickening that extends along the long axis of the aorta without evidence of intimal flap or penetrating ulcer; on unenhanced CT, the area of wall thickening frequently shows increased attenuation caused by acute hemorrhage (Fig. 3). Penetrating ulcers typically appear as focal ulcers with adjacent subintimal hematoma in the middle or distal third of the descending thoracic aorta; they rarely occur in the ascending aorta or arch due to the relative sparing of these areas by atherosclerosis. In patients with aortic rupture, portable chest radiographs show focal (Fig. 4) or diffuse (Fig. 5) aortic widening associated with pleural effusion representing hemothorax.

The radiographic findings of pneumonia consist of parenchymal opacification that is typically focal but may be multifocal (Fig. 6); associated infiltration of the adjacent chest wall suggests specific infections such as actinomycosis, nocardiosis, blastomycosis, aspergillosis, and tuberculosis (Fig. 7). Empyema manifests radiographically as a pleural-based mass with obtuse angles relative to the chest wall (Fig. 8A); on contrast-enhanced CT evaluation, a loculated pleural effusion associated with enhancement and thickening of separated visceral and parietal pleurae (split pleura sign) may be seen (Fig. 8B).

Radiographic detection of Pancoast tumors in early stages is often problematic because of obscuration of the lung apex by overlying ribs and

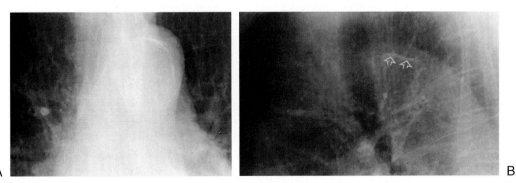

A   B

FIG. 1. Displacement of calcified intimal plaque indicative of type B dissection in a 79-year-old woman. **A** and **B:** Posteroanterior and lateral radiographs demonstrate medial and inferior (*arrows*) displacement of intimal calcification, respectively.

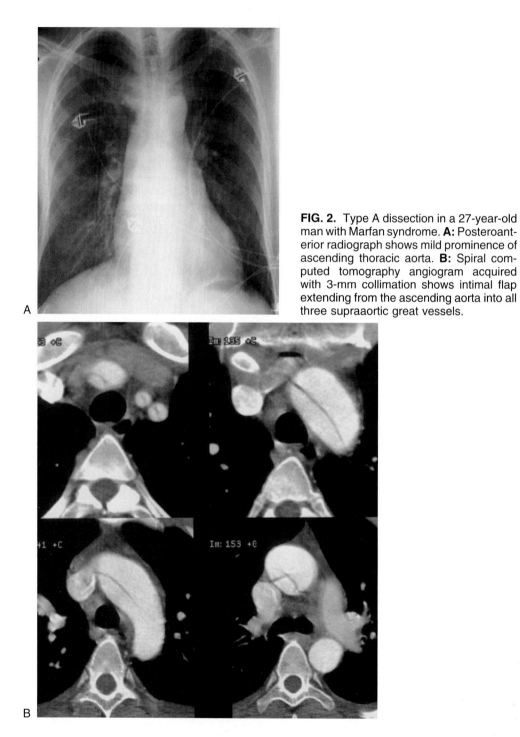

FIG. 2. Type A dissection in a 27-year-old man with Marfan syndrome. **A:** Posteroanterior radiograph shows mild prominence of ascending thoracic aorta. **B:** Spiral computed tomography angiogram acquired with 3-mm collimation shows intimal flap extending from the ascending aorta into all three supraaortic great vessels.

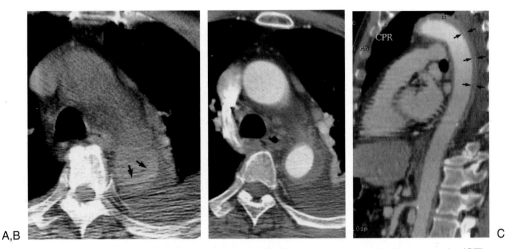

A,B   C

FIG. 3. Intramural hematoma in a 68-year-old man. **A:** Noncontrast computed tomography (CT) scan obtained with 10-mm collimation shows crescent of high attenuation (*arrows*) along the posterolateral aspect of the proximal descending aorta consistent with acute hemorrhage. **B:** Contrast-enhanced 3-mm collimation CT image at the same level shows circumferential mural thickening of the proximal descending aorta, most prominently involving the posterolateral wall. The ascending aorta is normal. **C:** Curved planar reformation of a spiral CT data set acquired with 3-mm collimation shows intramural hematoma (*arrows*) extending along the long axis of the descending thoracic aorta.

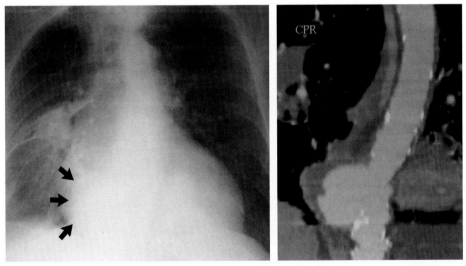

A   B

FIG. 4. Leaking pseudoaneurysm arising from penetrating ulcer in an 88-year-old man. **A:** Poster-oanterior radiograph shows mass (*arrows*) in the right retrocardiac region associated with a small right pleural effusion and pseudotumor in the major fissure. **B:** Curved planar reformation of a spiral computed tomography data set acquired with 3-mm collimation shows a pseudoaneurysm involving the right lateral aspect of the descending thoracic aorta associated with an adjacent hematoma.

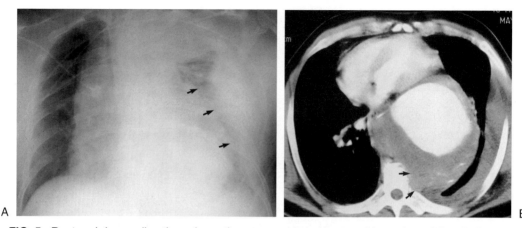

FIG. 5. Ruptured descending thoracic aortic aneurysm in a 43-year-old cocaine addict. **A:** Portable chest radiograph shows marked dilatation of the descending thoracic aorta (*arrows*) associated with moderate-sized loculated left pleural effusion and marked mediastinal shift to the right. The patient subsequently died in the operating room. **B:** Contrast-enhanced computed tomography scan obtained with 10-mm collimation 5 hours before **(A)** shows a descending thoracic aortic aneurysm measuring 12 cm in diameter. Close application of the posterior wall of the aneurysm to the spine with lateral draping of the aneurysm around the vertebral body (*arrows*) (draped aorta sign) is consistent with leakage into the pleural cavity resulting in hemothorax.

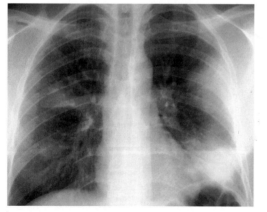

FIG. 6. Multilobar pneumococcal pneumonia in a 33-year-old man. Posteroanterior radiograph shows multiple bilateral, peripheral wedge-shaped parenchymal opacities.

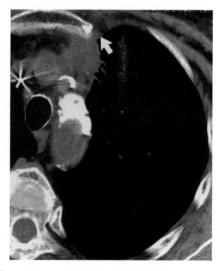

FIG. 7. Actinomycosis in an 87-year-old woman. Computed tomography scan obtained with 7-mm collimation shows soft tissue mass in the medial aspect left upper lobe extending into the mediastinum and chest wall (*arrow*).

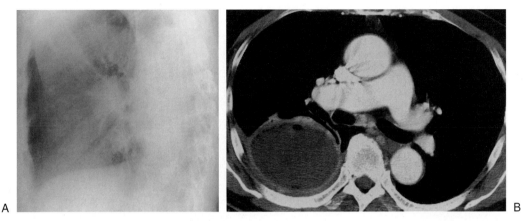

A   B

FIG. 8. Tuberculous empyema in a 77-year-old man. **A:** Lateral radiograph shows an elliptical pleural-based mass in the posterior hemithorax. **B:** Contrast-enhanced computed tomography scan obtained with 7-mm collimation shows a fluid collection bordered by thickened, enhancing visceral and parietal pleurae. The presence of a small amount of air in a nondependent region indicates the presence of a bronchopleural fistula.

clavicle and uncertain clinical significance of "apical pleural thickening" (Fig. 9). To minimize the risk of overlooking Pancoast tumors, asymmetric apical pleural thickening should always precipitate further evaluation by correlation with clinical symptoms and comparison with prior films.

Characteristic radiographic findings of esoph-

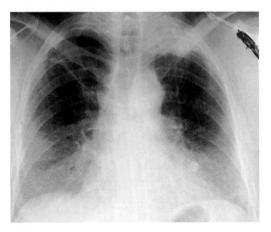

FIG. 9. Pancoast tumor in a 45-year-old man with symptoms of left shoulder and arm pain. Expiratory chest radiograph shows an asymmetric opacification of the left apex without associated bony destruction. Bullae are present in the right apical region.

ageal perforation consist of mediastinal emphysema, basilar consolidation, and pleural effusion with laterality dependent on location of the rupture site (Fig. 10). Extraluminal contrast extravasation on esophagography is diagnostic.

V. SENSITIVITY AND SPECIFICITY

Helical CT, TEE, and MRI detection of aortic dissection have equivalent sensitivities and specificities in the 95% to 100% range (2).

VI. DIFFERENTIAL DIAGNOSIS

Normal radiographic findings in a patient presenting with acute chest pain require consideration and either clinical or radiologic exclusion of potentially lethal entities such as aortic dissection, pulmonary embolism, and esophageal perforation. Ischemic heart disease is a common cause of acute chest pain; this entity has not been discussed because it often has no radiographic correlates and is diagnosed on the basis of biochemical and ECG findings.

VII. PITFALLS

Prospective diagnosis of possible aortic dissection on the basis of radiographic findings

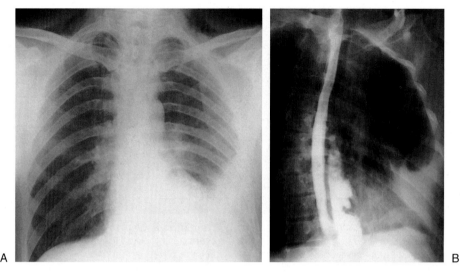

A   B

FIG. 10. Ruptured esophagus in a 40-year-old man after vomiting. **A:** Posteroanterior radiograph shows extensive mediastinal and subcutaneous emphysema associated with left pleural effusion. **B:** Oblique view from water-soluble contrast esophagram shows leakage of contrast along the left lateral aspect of the distal esophagus.

is made in only about one-fourth of affected patients, and completely normal radiographs occur in approximately 15% of patients (3). Because of the unreliability of radiographs, further evaluation using cross-sectional modalities should always be performed in patients in whom there exists a high clinical suspicion of aortic dissection. Similarly, esophagography should always be performed in all patients suspected of having esophageal rupture because chest radiographs are normal in approximately 10% (4).

VIII. REFERENCES

1. Spittell P, Spittell J, Joyce J, et al. Clinical features and differential diagnosis of aortic dissection: experience with 236 cases (1980 through 1990). *Mayo Clin Proc* 1993;68:642–651.
2. Sommer T, Fehske W, Holzknecht N, et al. Aortic dissection: a comparative study of diagnosis with spiral CT, multiplanar transesophageal echocardiography, and MR imaging. *Radiology* 1996;199:347–352.
3. Luker G, Glazer H, Eagar G, Gutierrez F, Sagel S. Aortic dissection: effect of prospective chest radiographic diagnosis on delay to definitive diagnosis. *Radiology* 1994; 193:813–819.
4. Henderson J, Peloquin A. Boerhaave revisited: spontaneous esophageal perforation as a diagnostic masquerader. *Am J Med* 1989;86:559–567.

7

Acute Shortness of Breath

Ann N. Leung

I. CLINICAL OVERVIEW

Acute shortness of breath (SOB) may be caused by a wide variety of cardiopulmonary diseases. Pulmonary embolism (PE) is the classic disease that presents with dyspnea of sudden onset, which is sometimes accompanied by hemoptysis and pleuritic chest pain. It is estimated that each year in the United States, PE occurs in more than 600,000 patients and causes up to 50,000 deaths. Recognized risk factors predisposing to PE include surgery involving general anesthesia for more than 30 minutes, injury or surgery involving the lower extremities or pelvis, congestive heart failure, prolonged immobility, pregnancy, cancer, and use of estrogen-containing compounds.

Pulmonary infection is the most common cause of dyspnea in young adults; patients typically present with associated symptoms of fever, cough, and occasionally, pleuritic chest pain. Pleural diseases such as pneumothorax and hemothorax are characterized by rapid onset; in the absence of an antecedent history of trauma, spontaneous pneumothorax should be suspected in tall, young men who suddenly develop dyspnea often accompanied by chest pain.

Pulmonary edema due to either left heart failure or overhydration (including renal failure) is one of the most common causes of acute SOB in elderly and hospitalized patients. Increased-permeability or injury-type pulmonary edema is discussed in the context of acute respiratory distress syndrome in Chapter 9.

Diffuse pulmonary hemorrhage is an uncommon but important cause of acute SOB and is discussed in greater depth in Chapter 8. In young adults, parenchymal hemorrhage typically occurs in association with an underlying collagen vascular disorder (systemic lupus erythematosus and Wegener's granulomatosis), Goodpasture's syndrome, or leukemia.

Acute eosinophilic pneumonia (AEP) is a rare disease of unknown etiology first described in 1989. Patients with this syndrome may be any age and typically present with an acute febrile illness and dyspnea, which can rapidly progress to hypoxic respiratory failure. Unlike other forms of eosinophilic lung disease, a raised peripheral eosinophil count is not present in the majority of patients. AEP responds rapidly to and is cured by corticosteroid therapy. Diagnosis requires an invasive procedure such as bronchoalveolar lavage to document the presence of lung eosinophilia.

Acute interstitial pneumonia, previously known as Hamman-Rich syndrome, is a form of idiopathic interstitial pneumonia that can present with acute and rapidly progressive SOB. In affected patients, who are usually middle aged or older, symptoms typically progress to respiratory failure and death.

Neoplastic diseases are an infrequent cause of acute SOB. Three manifestations of malignant disease that may include dyspnea as a prominent symptom are obstructive atelectasis or pneumonia, lymphangitic carcinomatosis (LC), and superior vena cava (SVC) syndrome. LC is an entity in which metastatic tumor growth occurs primarily in the lymphatics of the lung parenchyma; the most commonly associated histology is adenocarcinoma. SVC syndrome may result from either compression or direct invasion of the great veins of the thoracic inlet by either lymphadenopathy or the primary tumor, which most commonly is small-cell carcinoma. In addition to dyspnea, most patients experience headache and on physical examination exhibit signs of facial or upper extremity swelling.

II. IMAGING STRATEGY

Chest radiographs are used as the initial imaging study to evaluate patients presenting with acute SOB. Workup for PE should be initiated if there is either a high clinical suspicion or if the extent of radiographic pleuroparenchymal disease is discordant with the degree of hypoxemia. Although imperfect as a screening procedure because of its high yield of nondiagnostic (intermediate and low probability) studies, ventilation/perfusion (V/Q) scintigraphy remains the initial study performed at most institutions. Use of helical computed tomographic (CT) pulmonary angiography as the initial screening test may be indicated in select patient populations (inpatients and those with chronic obstructive pulmonary disease or focal radiographic consolidation) who are recognized to have a high rate of nondiagnostic V/Q studies (1). Pulmonary angiography remains the imaging gold standard for detection of PE.

III. TECHNIQUE

Optimized helical CT pulmonary angiography consists of a thin-collimation (3 mm) volumetric study acquired using high injection rates of nonionic contrast (4 to 5 mL/s of 300 mg iodine/mL) and reconstructed with overlapping increments (2 mm). CT evaluation should extend from the level of the aortic arch to 1 cm below the level of the inferior pulmonary veins; using a pitch of 2, 18 cm of coverage can be obtained with a 30-second breath-hold. Scan acquisition timed to the optimal phase of arterial opacification is achieved by performance of an initial test bolus of 10 mL of contrast; scanning delay is set to the earliest time of peak contrast opacification in the main pulmonary artery as measured on a generated time-density curve and typically ranges from 6 to 12 seconds. Including the timing bolus, the total volume of contrast

administered is 130 mL. Scanning from a caudad to cephalad direction can help minimize motion artifacts in patients unable to maintain apnea throughout the scanning period.

IV. FINDINGS

Pulmonary embolism is found in association with radiographic abnormalities in approximately 85% of cases. The most common findings are usually nonspecific and consist of atelectasis or parenchymal areas of increased opacity and pleural effusions. Relatively more specific findings include regional oligemia (Westermark sign); peripheral, wedge-shaped, pleural-based opacities (Hampton hump); and enlargement of central pulmonary arteries (Fleischner sign). Although unusual, extensive parenchymal disease should never exclude PE, particularly if the patient has known risk factors or is hypoxic (Fig. 1). Emboli on helical CT angiography manifest as intraarterial filling defects that may be partially or completely occlusive (Fig. 2).

Although considerable overlap of the radiographic patterns of pneumonia caused by different infectious agents occurs, broad generalizations regarding the appearance and distribution of parenchymal involvement are sometimes

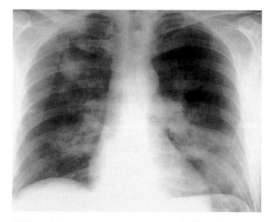

FIG. 1. Massive pulmonary embolism in a 45-year-old man who required thrombolytic therapy for persistent hypotension. A portable radiograph at the time of presentation shows patchy, bilateral parenchymal opacities.

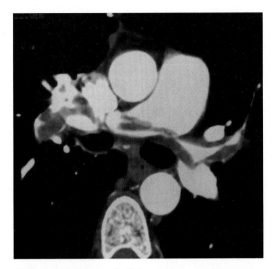

FIG. 2. Saddle emboli in a 48-year-old woman with lung cancer. Spiral computed tomographic pulmonary angiogram obtained with 3-mm collimation shows multiple tubular filling defects in the central pulmonary arteries.

helpful in specifying an etiologic group. An alveolar pattern with consolidation as its most severe form is the most common manifestation of bacterial pneumonia; cavitation within areas of consolidation (necrotizing pneumonia) suggest gram-negative and anaerobic organisms (Fig. 3A), *Staphylococcus aureus* and *Mycobacterium tuberculosis*. Solitary or multiple, nodular or masslike opacities with or without cavitation are manifestations of septic emboli, bacterial lung abscess, granulomatous infections such as tuberculosis and regional mycoses (Fig. 3B), and opportunistic fungal infections including aspergillus (Fig. 3C) if the patient is neutropenic or on immunosuppressive therapy. Fine reticular, reticulonodular, or ground-glass patterns of disease are often seen in viral, mycoplasma (Fig. 3D), and *Pneumocystis carinii* infections at presentation; the distribution of these "atypical" pneumonias also differs from bacterial and fungal infections in that parenchymal involvement may be diffuse and bilateral even in early stages. A miliary pattern consists of 1- to 3-mm nodules in a diffuse, bilateral distribution and indicates hematogenous dissemination of mycobacterial or fungal organisms (Fig. 3E).

Infrequently, the differential diagnosis of pulmonary infection may be narrowed to a short list of causative organisms because of the presence of a specific associated radiographic finding. The bulging fissure sign refers to expansion of a consolidated lobe with convex displacement of its fissure and is found in association with exudative pneumonias caused by Klebsiella (Fig. 4), *M. tuberculosis*, and pneumococci. Chest wall involvement resulting in pain or radiographically apparent rib destruction may occur with actinomycosis, nocardiosis, blastomycosis, aspergillosis, and tuberculosis.

The parenchymal abnormalities associated with cardiogenic and fluid overload pulmonary edema are diffuse, bilateral and symmetric; any unexplained deviation from this distribution suggests the presence of other or coexistent processes. Regional disruptions of the normal pulmonary vascular circulation can result in patchy or asymmetric distributions; emphysema (Fig. 5A), mitral regurgitation (Fig. 5B), and unilateral dependent positioning (Fig. 5C) are common causes for atypical patterns of pulmonary edema. Cardiomegaly, vascular redistribution, interlobular septal thickening (Kerley lines), subpleural edema, and pleural effusions are associated findings that may help to indicate the correct diagnosis.

The radiographic manifestations of AEP consist of a diffuse, fine reticular pattern associated with hazy parenchymal opacification and, occasionally, effusions (Fig. 6); CT findings consist predominantly of ground-glass opacities that may be focal or diffuse in distribution. The radiographic manifestations of acute interstitial pneumonia are progressive consolidation usually occurring in a bilateral, symmetric, and predominantly basilar distribution (Fig. 7A); on high-resolution CT, diffuse consolidation is seen associated with scattered or diffuse ground-glass opacities (Fig. 7B).

Although segmental or lobar pneumonias are often accompanied by some degree of atelectasis, the presence of a central mass (Fig. 8, lack of air bronchograms in the atelectatic, consolidated lung, and persistence or recurrence of findings after appropriate therapy should always precipitate performance of CT or bronchoscopy to ex-

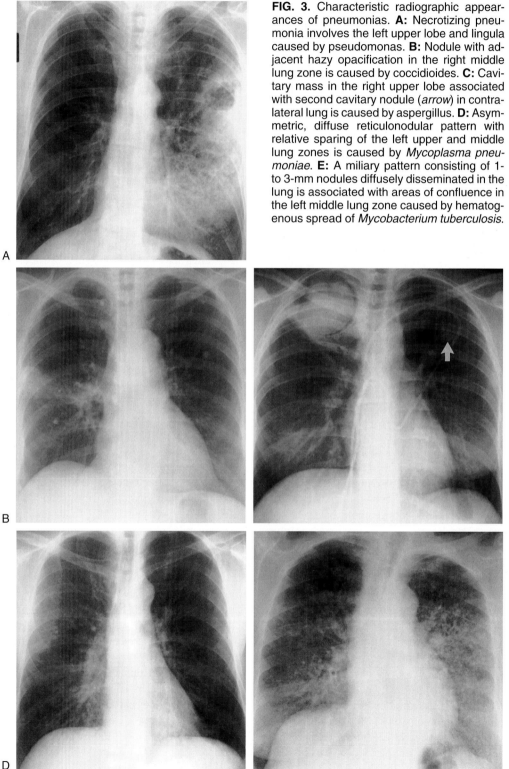

FIG. 3. Characteristic radiographic appearances of pneumonias. **A:** Necrotizing pneumonia involves the left upper lobe and lingula caused by pseudomonas. **B:** Nodule with adjacent hazy opacification in the right middle lung zone is caused by coccidioides. **C:** Cavitary mass in the right upper lobe associated with second cavitary nodule (*arrow*) in contralateral lung is caused by aspergillus. **D:** Asymmetric, diffuse reticulonodular pattern with relative sparing of the left upper and middle lung zones is caused by *Mycoplasma pneumoniae*. **E:** A miliary pattern consisting of 1- to 3-mm nodules diffusely disseminated in the lung is associated with areas of confluence in the left middle lung zone caused by hematogenous spread of *Mycobacterium tuberculosis*.

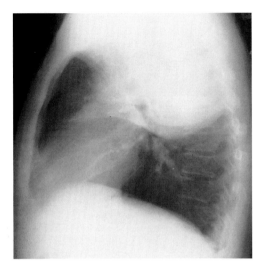

FIG. 4. Bulging fissure sign in a 60-year-old man with Klebsiella (Friedlander's) pneumonia. Lateral radiograph shows consolidation of the right upper lobe with an inferior convexity of major fissure.

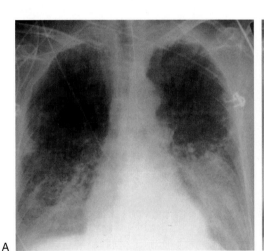

A

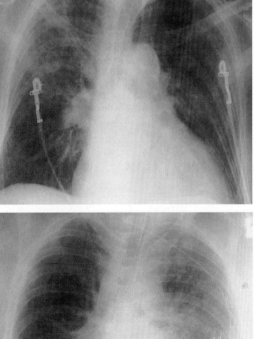

B

FIG. 5. Atypical radiographic patterns of pulmonary edema. **A:** Relative sparing of bilateral upper lobes is seen in a 56-year-old man with severe centrilobular (smoking-induced) emphysema. **B:** Focal area of greater severity involves the right upper lobe in a 78-year-old man with documented mitral regurgitation. **C:** Asymmetric left-sided predominance is seen in a 67-year-old man immediately after right hemipelvectomy for chondrosarcoma.

C

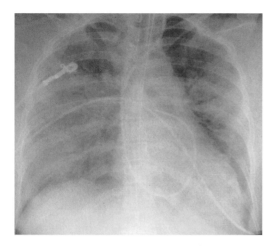

FIG. 6. Acute eosinophilic pneumonia in a 45-year-old woman diagnosed with bronchoalveolar lavage. Portable radiograph shows diffuse, homogeneous opacification of bilateral lungs.

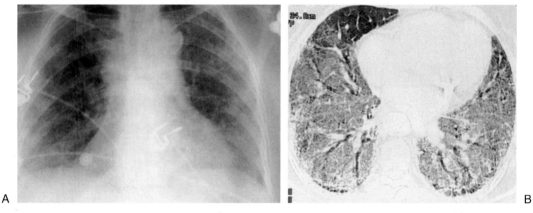

A   B

FIG. 7. Acute interstitial pneumonia in a 72-year-old woman resulting in death. **A:** Anteroposterior chest radiograph shows diffuse, fine reticular pattern. **B:** A 1-mm collimation computed tomography scan shows diffuse ground-glass opacities associated with microcystic changes in the peripheral aspects of the posterior lower lobes.

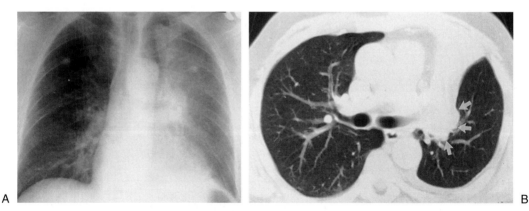

A   B

FIG. 8. Obstructive atelectasis in a 58-year-old man with bronchogenic carcinoma. **A:** Posteroanterior radiograph shows a left hilar mass associated with truncation of the left upper lobe bronchus and upper lobe atelectasis. **B:** Corresponding computed tomography scan obtained with 7-mm collimation shows an atelectatic left upper lobe without air bronchograms and a convex contour of displaced fissure (*arrows*) in the hilar region caused by the obstructive mass.

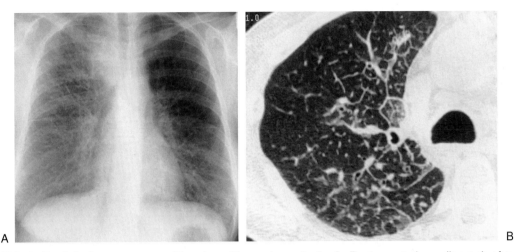

A   B

FIG. 9. Radiologic appearance of lymphangitic carcinomatosis. **A:** Posteroanterior radiograph of a 44-year-old woman with adenocarcinoma of unknown origin shows asymmetric distribution of diffuse reticular pattern associated with Kerley B lines and right paratracheal lymphadenopathy. **B:** A 1-mm collimation computed tomography scan targeted to the right lung of a 61-year-old man with colonic carcinoma shows nodular thickening of interlobular septa associated with patchy areas of ground-glass attenuation representing focal edema.

clude a central obstructive lesion. The radiographic findings of LC consist of a reticular or reticulonodular pattern associated with Kerley B lines; coexisting lymphadenopathy and a focal or asymmetric distribution are distinguishing features that can differentiate LC from pulmonary edema, the entity for which it is often mistaken (Fig. 9A). The high-resolution CT appearance of LC is highly characteristic: nodular thickening is identified along interlobular septa and bronchovascular bundles (Fig. 9B). Patients with SVC syndrome typically have radiographic evidence of a mediastinal mass; contrast-enhanced CT scan is diagnostic and can allow direct visualization of the cause and point of obstruction (Fig. 10).

V. SENSITIVITY AND SPECIFICITY

Reported sensitivity and specificity of helical CT pulmonary angiography for detection of PE range from 82% to 94% and 78% to 95%, respectively (1–3). According to results from the Prospective Investigation of Pulmonary Embolism Diagnosis (PIOPED) trial (4), positive (high-, intermediate-, and low-probability) V/Q studies had a sensitivity of 98% and specificity of 10% for PE; reported sensitivity and specificity for high-probability V/Q scans were 41% and 97%, respectively.

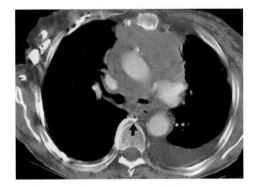

FIG. 10. Superior vena cava (SVC) syndrome in a 65-year-old woman with poorly differentiated non–small-cell carcinoma. Computed tomography scan obtained with 7-mm collimation shows extensive soft tissue infiltration of the mediastinum with complete obliteration and nonvisualization of the SVC. Collateral vessels are present in the chest wall with dense opacification of the azygos vein (*arrow*).

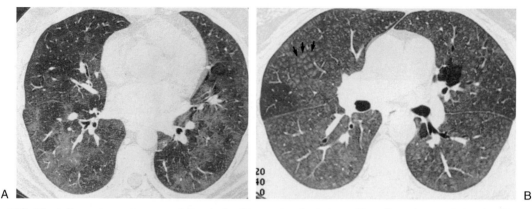

FIG. 11. Inflammatory diseases characterized by acute shortness of breath and normal chest radiograph. **A:** A 1-mm collimation computed tomography (CT) scan of a 45-year-old man with *Pneumocystis carinii* pneumonia who was receiving corticosteroid therapy shows diffuse ground-glass opacities. **B:** A 1-mm collimation CT scan of a 55-year-old bird fancier with extrinsic allergic alveolitis shows diffuse ground-glass attenuation associated with centrilobular nodules (*arrows*).

VI. DIFFERENTIAL DIAGNOSIS

Acute shortness of breath in a patient with a normal radiograph significantly narrows the differential diagnosis to entities that either impair oxygenation by obstruction of blood or air flow or cause subtle and diffuse infiltration of the lung parenchyma not detectable on radiographs. Normal radiographs are found in 12% to 16% of patients with angiographically proven PE. Exacerbations of asthma and chronic obstructive pulmonary disease are common causes of acute SOB; radiographs taken during the time of acute exacerbation in both of these obstructive lung diseases are of limited value because they typically show no change from the preexacerbation state. Mild to moderate SOB in patients with normal chest radiographs may occasionally be a presenting symptom of a diffuse, inflammatory parenchymal process of insufficient density to create radiographically apparent abnormalities. Normal radiographs are a recognized manifestation of infections caused by *P. carinii* pneumonia and viruses, such as cytomegalovirus; ground-glass opacities sometimes present in a geographic distribution are the most common high-resolution CT findings of *P. carinii* pneumonia (Fig. 11A). Extrinsic allergic alveolitis is a form of immunologically mediated lung disease caused by exposure to a variety of organic antigens; high-resolution CT scans of patients with extrinsic allergic alveolitis and a normal chest radiograph are reported to demonstrate patchy ground-glass opacities with associated centrilobular nodules (Fig. 11B).

VII. PITFALLS

Lack of visualization of subsegmental pulmonary arteries is the greatest limitation of helical CT pulmonary angiography. Because emboli isolated to subsegmental or smaller pulmonary arterial branches are the only manifestation of PE in 6% to 30% of cases (4,5), widespread adoption of helical CT pulmonary angiography as the initial screening procedure is unlikely to occur until improvements in scanner technology enable visualization and evaluation of more distal pulmonary arteries.

VIII. REFERENCES

1. Mayo JR, Remy-Jardin M, Muller NL, et al. Pulmonary embolism: prospective comparison of spiral CT with ventilation-perfusion scintigraphy. *Radiology* 1997;205:447–452.
2. Remy-Jardin M, Remy J, Deschildre F, et al. Diagnosis of pulmonary embolism with spiral CT: comparison with

pulmonary angiography and scintigraphy. *Radiology* 1996;200:699–706.

3. Van Rossum AB, Pattynama PMT, Ton ERTA, et al. Pulmonary embolism: validation of spiral CT angiography in 149 patients. *Radiology* 1996;201:467–470.

4. The PIOPED Investigators. Value of the ventilation/perfusion scan in acute pulmonary embolism: results of the Prospective Investigation of Pulmonary Embolism Diagnosis. *JAMA* 1990;263:2753–2759.

5. Goodman LR, Lipchik RJ. Diagnosis of acute pulmonary embolism: time for a new approach. *Radiology* 1996;199:25–27.

8

Hemoptysis

Ann N. Leung

I. CLINICAL OVERVIEW

Hemoptysis is one of the most alarming symptoms for which a patient seeks medical attention. For purposes of management, hemoptysis is traditionally divided into two categories: massive and submassive. Massive hemoptysis (more than 600 mL/24 h) represents a life-threatening condition; although exsanguination is rare, mortality can result from asphyxiation caused by aspirated blood interfering with gas exchange.

In developed countries, the most common causes of massive hemoptysis are bronchiectasis, mycetoma, and bronchogenic carcinoma. Active pulmonary tuberculosis, usually cavitary in nature, is the single most important cause in third-world populations. In the vast majority of cases, bronchial arteries and systemic collaterals from axillary, intercostal, internal mammary, subclavian, and phrenic arteries are the source of bleeding. Angiography with bronchial arterial embolization has been an effective method to achieve primary control of bleeding and is successful in 84% to 100% of cases (1).

Infections are the most common cause of submassive hemoptysis in younger adults. Patients with mycetomas and postinfectious complications such as bronchiectasis and broncholithiasis more commonly present to medical attention because of expectoration of small amounts of blood rather than massive hemoptysis. Cystic fibrosis is the prototypical disease in which underlying bronchiectasis associated with chronic inflammation results in frequent bouts of hemoptysis. Broncholithiasis is an uncommon complication of granulomatous diseases characterized by calcified peribronchial nodes that either erode into or cause significant distortion of an adjacent bronchus.

Neoplastic disease is a common cause of submassive hemoptysis in older patients. Parenchymal cavitation and central tracheobronchial location are the two characteristics of tumors that predispose to expectoration of blood and are frequently seen in association with squamous and carcinoid histologies, respectively. Central tracheobronchial tumors may also be caused by endobronchial metastases, which most commonly arise from primary tumors in the breast, kidney, gastrointestinal tract, and skin (melanoma). Rarely, vascular tumors such as Kaposi's sarcoma and angiosarcoma may cause hemoptysis.

Pulmonary embolism (PE) is an important entity that should always be considered in the differential diagnosis of hemoptysis; dyspnea and chest pain are associated symptoms that often alert to the correct diagnosis.

Diffuse pulmonary hemorrhage (DPH) is a syndrome caused by a heterogeneous group of disorders clinically characterized by dyspnea, hemoptysis, and anemia. DPH may be seen in association with predisposing medical conditions such as systemic lupus erythematosus, Wegener's granulomatosis, Goodpasture's syndrome, and bone marrow transplantation, or it may occur in isolation as idiopathic pulmonary hemosiderosis, an entity that typically affects children less than 10 years of age or boys above the age of 10. Hemorrhage is the most common noninfectious cause of radiographic parenchymal opacities in leukemia and typically occurs in patients with platelet counts less than 50,000 cells/μL. DPH rarely occurs as a complication of anticoagulant therapy.

Elevation of pulmonary venous pressure is a recognized cause of hemoptysis, typically occurring in patients with mitral stenosis and occasionally cardiogenic pulmonary edema. Hemoptysis is the presenting symptom in approximately 10% of patients with pulmonary arteriovenous malformations (AVM) (1). Aortobronchial fistula is a rare and potentially lethal condition associated with hemoptysis. Fistula formation typically develops between a thoracic aortic aneurysm or postsurgical pseudoaneurysm and the left lung with upper and lower lobe bronchi reported to be involved with equal frequency. Prospective diagnosis is difficult because the fistulous communication is rarely demonstrated on either helical computed tomography (CT) or conventional angiography.

II. IMAGING STRATEGY

Chest radiographs should be the initial imaging study obtained in a patient presenting with hemoptysis. Radiographic evaluation of patients with massive hemoptysis occasionally reveals the cause of bleeding but is more often nonlocalizing; in this emergent setting, bronchoscopy is the procedure of choice to localize the bleeding site and to guide further therapeutic procedures.

In patients with submassive hemoptysis and focal radiographic findings, CT scanning may be used to better characterize the abnormalities and guide the most efficacious selection of biopsy sites and procedures. CT and bronchoscopy are complementary procedures in the evaluation of patients with submassive hemoptysis and a normal chest radiograph; which diagnostic test is initially performed largely depends on individual physician preference. Comparative advantages of CT over bronchoscopy are detection of bronchiectasis and radiographically occult peripheral cancers; comparative disadvantages are an inability to biopsy and insensitive mucosal evaluation resulting in missed diagnoses of bronchitis and squamous metaplasia (2).

III. TECHNIQUE

An optimized CT protocol for evaluation of hemoptysis enables visualization of fine paren-

chymal structures as required for detection of bronchiectasis along with assessment of the entire central tracheobronchial tree down to the segmental bronchi level. Thin-section (1- to 2-mm) images should be obtained every 10 mm from the thoracic inlet to the carina; a volumetric acquisition of 3- to 5-mm images is then obtained through the central airways to the level of basilar segmental bronchi; and finally, thin-section images are obtained every 10 mm from the inferior level of the volumetric study to the lung bases. Intravenous contrast may be used when indicated by radiographic findings to further assess the mediastinum or hila.

IV. FINDINGS

Infectious agents commonly associated with hemoptysis such as *Mycobacterium tuberculosis* (Fig. 1) and gram-negative organisms can often be recognized on radiographs because of their shared predisposition for lung destruction, resulting in cavitary or necrotizing pneumonias. A distribution involving the apical or posterior segments of the upper lobe or superior segment of the lower lobe should always raise concern for postprimary tuberculosis.

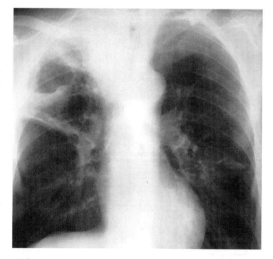

FIG. 1. Tuberculosis in a 36-year-old man. Posteroanterior radiograph shows a large cavity in the right upper lobe associated with right paratracheal lymphadenopathy.

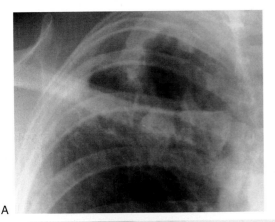

A

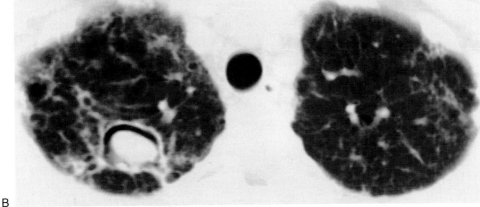

B

FIG. 2. Aspergilloma in a 33-year-old woman. **A:** Directed view shows a nodule in a right upper lobe cavity. **B:** Computed tomography scan obtained with 7-mm collimation shows an intracavitary nodule occupying a dependent position; reticular opacities with associated architectural distortion in upper lobes represent fibrosis.

A mycetoma represents colonization of a preexisting cavity by aspergillus. Radiographically, an aspergilloma appears as a roughly spherical nodule or mass separated by a crescent-shaped lucency from the adjacent cavity wall (Fig. 2A); CT features consist of a mobile intracavitary nodule or mass that gravitates to the dependent position on prone and supine images (Fig. 2B).

Bronchiectasis is frequently undetected or underestimated on chest radiographs; in late stages, the characteristic findings consist of air–fluid levels within ''cysts'' (ectatic bronchi en face) arranged in lines or grapelike clusters (Fig. 3). On thin-section CT, bronchiectasis is diagnosed on the basis of bronchoarterial diameter ratio greater than 1, lack of normal peripheral tapering of bronchi, and visualization of bronchi with 1 cm of costal pleura (Fig. 4). The radiologic findings of broncholithiasis consist of

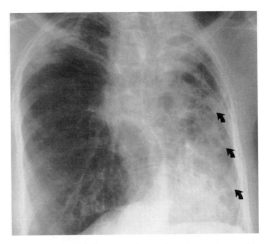

FIG. 3. Postinfectious bronchiectasis in a 21-year-old woman with a history of childhood tuberculosis. Posteroanterior radiograph shows marked volume loss of left lung, which contains multiple ''cystic'' spaces, some containing air–fluid levels (*arrows*).

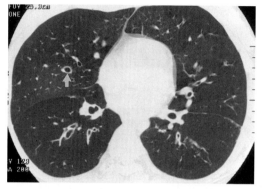

FIG. 4. Radiographically occult bronchiectasis in a 16-year-old girl. Computed tomography scan obtained with 1-mm collimation shows several bronchi with thickened walls and luminal size greater than accompanying pulmonary artery (signet ring sign) (*arrow*).

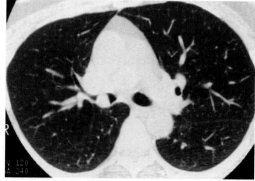

FIG. 6. Carcinoid tumor in a 51-year-old woman. Computed tomography scan obtained with 1-mm collimation shows a well-defined nodule in the lumen of the right mainstem bronchus.

calcified peribronchial nodes that are sometimes associated with segmental or lobar atelectasis, obstructive pneumonitis, or branching opacities in a ''V'' or ''Y'' configuration (obstructive bronchocele).

Neoplastic diseases most commonly manifest as nodules or masses with or without associated cavitation (Fig. 5); central lesions (Fig. 6) occasionally result in postobstructive atelectasis or pneumonitis. Vascular tumors such as Kaposi's sarcoma and angiosarcoma may manifest radiographically as poorly defined nodular opacities; on thin-section CT, pulmonary nodules are seen associated with adjacent areas of ground-glass attenuation (CT halo sign) representing hemorrhage (Fig. 7).

The radiologic findings of PE are discussed in Chapter 7. Clinical, radiographic, and scintigraphic findings of PE may occasionally be mimicked by pulmonary infarction caused by the use of crack cocaine (3) (Fig. 8). This entity

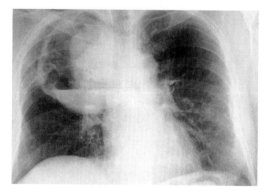

FIG. 5. Squamous cell carcinoma in a 61-year-old man. Posteroanterior radiograph shows a large cavitary mass containing air–fluid level in the right upper lobe.

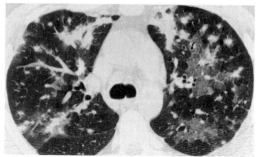

FIG. 7. Kaposi's sarcoma in a 42-year-old man with acquired immunodeficiency syndrome. Computed tomography scan obtained with 1-mm collimation shows multiple, irregularly marginated nodules scattered throughout both lungs associated with areas of ground-glass attenuation representing hemorrhage.

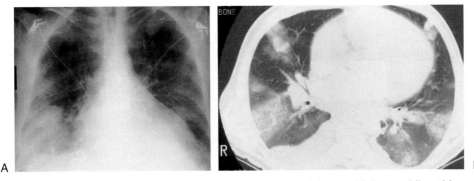

A   B

FIG. 8. Cocaine-induced parenchymal infarction in a 50-year-old man with known idiopathic cardiomyopathy. **A:** Anteroposterior radiograph shows patchy bilateral parenchymal consolidation involving bilateral middle and lower lung zones. **B:** A 7-mm collimation computed tomography scan shows multiple peripheral areas of wedge-shaped consolidation that on biopsy were found to represent bland infarcts.

is typically seen in younger patients and is believed to arise from intense vasoconstriction of the pulmonary vasculature resulting in anoxic cell damage and alveolar hemorrhage and edema (3).

The radiographic findings of DPH depend on the severity of parenchymal hemorrhage and may vary from normal to dense consolidation in any distribution, of which bilateral and diffuse is the most typical (Fig. 9). Rapidity of onset is a

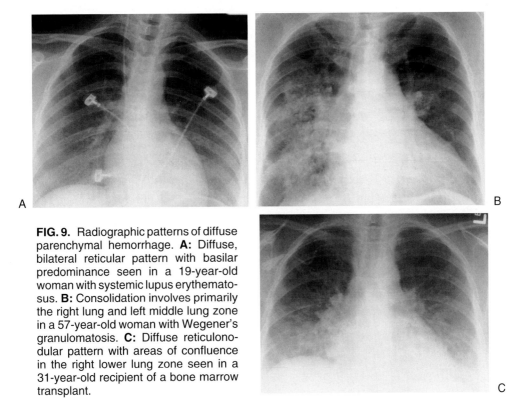

A   B

FIG. 9. Radiographic patterns of diffuse parenchymal hemorrhage. **A:** Diffuse, bilateral reticular pattern with basilar predominance seen in a 19-year-old woman with systemic lupus erythematosus. **B:** Consolidation involves primarily the right lung and left middle lung zone in a 57-year-old woman with Wegener's granulomatosis. **C:** Diffuse reticulonodular pattern with areas of confluence in the right lower lung zone seen in a 31-year-old recipient of a bone marrow transplant.

C

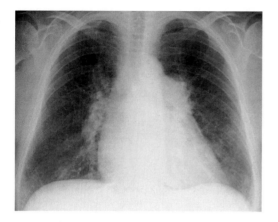

FIG. 10. Mitral stenosis and pulmonary artery hypertension in a 46-year-old woman with a history of rheumatic heart disease. Posteroanterior radiograph shows prominence of left atrial appendage and double density along the right cardiac margin consistent with left atrial enlargement; associated dilatation of the central pulmonary arteries is consistent with pulmonary artery hypertension.

characteristic feature of hemorrhagic disorders. Within 2 to 3 days of the acute bleed, air space consolidation is gradually replaced by a reticular pattern as blood is absorbed into the interstitium; the radiograph returns to normal in 1 to 2 weeks if bleeding does not recur.

Radiographs of patients with mitral stenosis demonstrate characteristic signs of enlargement of the left atrium; associated enlargement of central pulmonary arteries and right-sided cardiac chambers may be present if secondary pulmonary arterial hypertension has developed (Fig. 10). Radiologic diagnosis of an AVM rests on identification of a parenchymal nodule or mass accompanied by supplying pulmonary artery(ies) and draining pulmonary vein(s), a task more easily and confidently accomplished with CT than with plain films (Fig. 11).

V. SENSITIVITY AND SPECIFICITY

Based on small clinical series (2,4), the sensitivity of CT and bronchoscopy for detection of cancers in patients presenting with hemoptysis

is approximately 100% and 80% to 85%, respectively. The discrepancy in results between the two modalities is attributable to cancers peripheral to the area assessable by bronchoscopy.

VI. DIFFERENTIAL DIAGNOSIS

The three most common conditions diagnosed in patients with submassive hemoptysis and a normal chest radiograph are bronchiectasis, bronchitis, and central tumor (2,5).

VII. PITFALLS

Despite investigation by both CT and bronchoscopy, in approximately one-third of all patients presenting with hemoptysis the cause is not identified (5). Prognosis for such patients diagnosed with cryptogenic or idiopathic hemoptysis is excellent, with 5-year survival rates ranging from 85% to 95% (1).

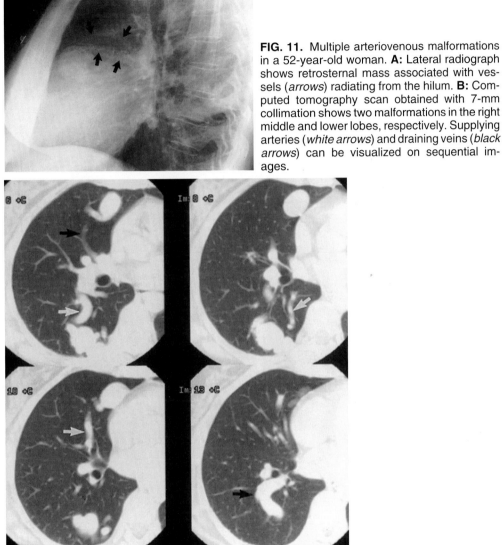

FIG. 11. Multiple arteriovenous malformations in a 52-year-old woman. **A:** Lateral radiograph shows retrosternal mass associated with vessels (*arrows*) radiating from the hilum. **B:** Computed tomography scan obtained with 7-mm collimation shows two malformations in the right middle and lower lobes, respectively. Supplying arteries (*white arrows*) and draining veins (*black arrows*) can be visualized on sequential images.

VIII. REFERENCES

1. Cahill BC, Ingbar DH. Massive hemoptysis–assessment and management. *Clin Chest Med* 1994;15:147–168.
2. Set PAK, Flower CDR, Smith IE, Cahn AP, Twentyman OP, Shneerson JM. Hemoptysis: comparative study of the role of CT and fiberoptic bronchoscopy. *Radiology* 1993;189:677–680.
3. Haim DY, Lippmann ML, Goldberg SK, Walkenstein MD. The pulmonary complications of crack cocaine–a comprehensive review. *Chest* 1995;107:233–240.
4. Naidich DP, Funt S, Ettenger NA, Arranda C. Hemoptysis: CT-bronchoscopic correlations in 58 cases. *Radiology* 1990;177:357–362.
5. Marshall TJ, Flower CDR, Jackson JE. The role of radiology in the investigation and management of patients with haemoptysis. *Clin Radiol* 1996;51:391–400.

9

Chest Imaging in the Intensive Care Unit

Ann N. Leung

I. CLINICAL OVERVIEW

Chest imaging has an important role in the noninvasive evaluation of ventilated patients in intensive care units (ICUs). Chest radiographs are used to assess the position of medical devices, to detect iatrogenic complications, and to assess the patient's cardiopulmonary status. Multiple outcome studies (1–3) have demonstrated that daily radiographs in this critically ill population will detect new or unsuspected findings that alter management in at least one-third of cases; yield of significant findings increases to one-half of cases when radiographs are prompted by a change in the clinical status of the patient (3).

Pneumothorax is a common complication in patients in the ICU and may develop from underlying lung disease or chest trauma or as a result of barotrauma from mechanical ventilation. Barotrauma is the most frequent cause of pneumomediastinum; elevated alveolar pressures cause alveolar rupture with dissection of gas along pulmonary interstitial pathways into the mediastinum. Raised pressure in pneumomediastinum can lead to rupture of the mediastinal pleura with subsequent pneumothorax and, rarely, hypotension caused by impaired venous return to the heart.

Atelectasis in ICU patients arises from a combination of factors including depression of mucociliary clearance, impairment of the cough reflex, reduction in lung surfactant, and passive atelectasis in the presence of pleural effusion or pneumothorax. The lobes most commonly affected by atelectasis in the ICU population are left lower (66%), right lower (22%), and right upper (11%).

Acute respiratory distress syndrome (ARDS), the clinical correlate of increased-permeability edema, is defined as a syndrome of inflammation and increased permeability associated with a constellation of clinical, physiologic, and radiologic abnormalities (4). ARDS is acute in onset and persistent, lasting days to weeks; associated with one or more known risk factors; and characterized by diffuse radiologic abnormalities and arterial hypoxia resistant to oxygen therapy alone (4). It is most commonly associated with sepsis syndrome, aspiration, primary pneumonia, multiple trauma, and fat embolism (4).

Ventilator-associated pneumonia (VAP) is a common complication affecting 9% to 20% of patients with respiratory failure (5). Oropharyngeal colonization with gram-negative bacilli frequently occurs in mechanically ventilated patients; secretions contaminated with microorganisms pooled just above the endotracheal tube (ETT) cuff are aspirated into the lower tracheobronchial tree and result in VAP.

II. IMAGING STRATEGY

Portable radiography is the technique of choice in evaluation of thoracic diseases and complications in ICU patients because of its accessibility, speed, low radiation dose, and relatively low cost. Computed tomography (CT) may be used in problematic cases in which either higher contrast resolution or cross-sectional anatomic display is needed.

III. TECHNIQUE

Although optimal evaluation of serial radiographs requires consistency in technical factors, this ideal is rarely attained. Consideration and comparison of film variables such as patient positioning, lung volumes, film-focal distance, and exposure factors with their respective, specific effects on radiographic appearance and diagnostic quality are important to differentiate true from artifactual changes in patient status. Computed radiography with its advantage of wider dynamic range ensures consistent image quality that is neither too dark nor too light.

IV. FINDINGS

A. Medical Devices

The tip of an ETT is ideally positioned 4 to 5 cm above the carina with the neck in a neutral position (Fig. 1); with neck flexion and extension, the tip can move 2 cm caudad and cephalad, respectively. The tip of a tracheostomy tube should be located one-half to two-thirds of the distance between the tracheal stoma and carina, at about the level of the third thoracic vertebral body. Although best assessed clinically, the balloon cuff of the ETT and tracheostomy tube should generally not be distended to a diameter greater than

the tracheal air column. Overdistention can result in ischemic necrosis and, ultimately, tracheal stenosis or malacia. Rupture, which usually involves the posterior membranous portion of the trachea, is an uncommon complication; early signs include marked enlargement of the balloon cuff, distal migration, and oblique orientation of the ETT toward the right.

Central venous catheters can be used for vascular access and monitoring of central venous pressure (CVP). Accurate CVP measurement requires the catheter tip to be positioned beyond the last venous valve, located distal to the anterior first rib. Cardiac complications such as arrhythmias and perforation are prevented by positioning of the catheter tip above the right atrium. Common aberrant catheter tip locations include the internal jugular, azygous, superior intercostal, contralateral subclavian, and axillary veins. A midsternal or left paravertebral location should raise suspicion of intraarterial placement (Fig. 2).

Tissue perforation is the most common, serious catheter-related complication; resulting injury depends on the anatomic location of the malpositioned catheter and may include pneumothorax, hemothorax (Fig. 3), mediastinal he-

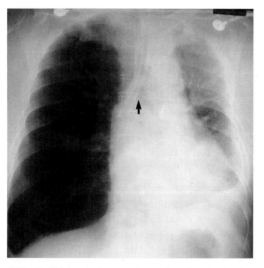

FIG. 1. Right mainstem bronchus intubation in an 86-year-old woman. Portable radiograph shows the tip of the endotracheal tube in the right mainstem bronchus (*arrow* points to tracheal carina) causing hyperinflation and atelectasis of the right and left lungs, respectively.

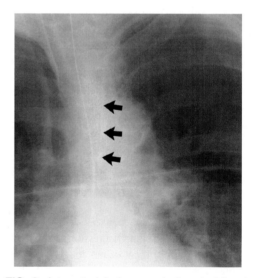

FIG. 2. Intraarterial placement of central line in a 57-year-old man. Slightly rotated (left anterior oblique) radiograph shows midline position of the left subclavian line tip (*arrow*), which is located in the descending thoracic aorta.

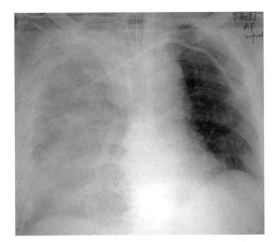

FIG. 3. Hemothorax resulting from line placement in a 68-year-old man. Portable radiograph shows the tip of the left subclavian catheter beyond the right lateral margin of the mediastinum; posteriorly layering right pleural effusion represents blood in the pleural cavity.

matoma, and cardiac perforation and tamponade. A curved catheter tip and a catheter tip directed against the wall of the superior vena cava (SVC) are radiographic signs that should prompt repositioning to avoid SVC perforation. Catheter fragmentation typically occurs in association with line insertion using a metallic needle introducer (Fig. 4) and can result in embolization

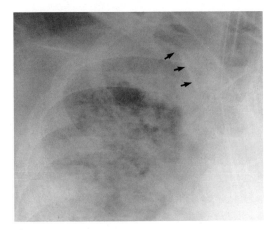

FIG. 4. Catheter fragment in a 24-year-old man after line removal. Directed radiograph shows catheter fragment (*arrows*) extending from the right subclavian to the brachiocephalic vein.

of fragments to the right side of the heart or pulmonary artery.

The tip of a Swan-Ganz catheter is ideally located in a large central pulmonary artery from where it can float distally to wedge when the balloon is inflated. Tip locations peripheral to proximal interlobar pulmonary arteries predispose to pulmonary infarction and pulmonary artery rupture with pseudoaneurysm formation (Fig. 5).

An intra-aortic balloon pump (IABP) is used in patients with cardiogenic shock and severely compromised left ventricular function to increase coronary artery perfusion and decrease cardiac afterload. The balloon is inflated only during diastole when it becomes radiographically visible as a sausage-shaped radiolucency. The radiopaque tip of an IABP is ideally located in the proximal descending thoracic aorta, distal to the origin of the left subclavian artery. More proximal and distal positions within the thoracic aorta may lead to obstruction of subclavian and renal arteries, respectively.

Chest tubes should be placed in anterosuperior and posteroinferior positions for drainage of pleural air and fluid collections, respectively. Side holes of chest tubes, marked by an interruption of the radiopaque identification line, should be positioned within the thoracic cavity, medial to the inner ribs. Accurate localization of chest tubes in subcutaneous, intrafissural, and intraparenchymal sites requires evaluation by lateral films and CT (Fig. 6).

The side hole and tip of a nasogastric tube are optimally located in the stomach. To minimize the risk of gastric aspiration, tips of feeding tubes should be positioned in the duodenum. Misplacement of enteral tubes into the tracheobronchial tree are predisposed in ICU patients with obtundation and poor cough reflexes and can result in lung perforation and aspiration of tube feedings, if unrecognized (Fig. 7).

All medical devices not clearly in an extrathoracic location require prompt identification and localization. Retained surgical instruments or sponges (Fig. 8A) and embolized catheters (Fig. 8B) are potentially serious complications in which patient morbidity may be decreased by early detection and retrieval.

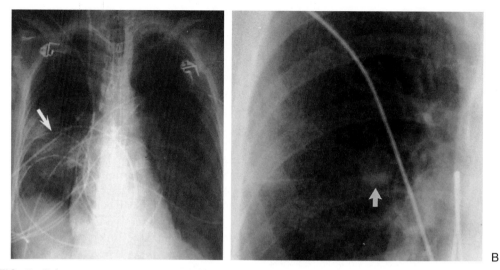

A   B

FIG. 5. Pulmonary artery rupture resulting from inflation of a Swan-Ganz catheter balloon in the peripheral pulmonary artery in a 70-year-old woman. **A:** Portable radiograph shows the tip of a Swan-Ganz catheter (*arrow*) peripheral to an interlobar artery; adjacent parenchymal opacification represents hemorrhage. **B:** Directed view obtained 10 days after **(A)** shows development of a well-circumscribed 2-cm nodule in the right upper lobe representing a pseudoaneurysm.

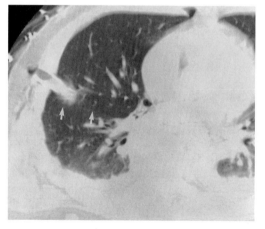

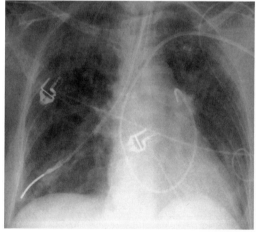

FIG. 6. Intraparenchymal location of a chest tube in a 37-year-old man. A computed tomography scan obtained with 3-mm collimation shows placement of the chest tube into the right middle lobe anterior to the major fissure (*arrows*). A small, anteromedial pneumothorax is associated.

FIG. 7. Placement of a feeding tube into the right lung of a 59-year-old woman. Portable radiograph shows the feeding tube coursing in the right tracheobronchial tree to terminate in the peripheral right lower lung.

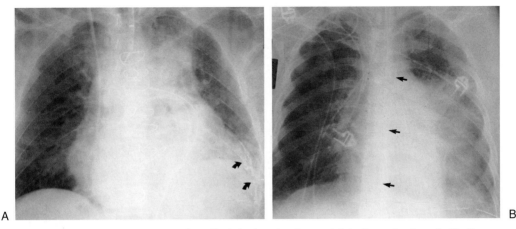

FIG. 8. Radiographic appearance of medical devices in aberrant, intrathoracic sites. **A:** Radiopaque threads mark a retained surgical sponge (*arrows*) in the inferior left hemithorax. **B:** Embolized guidewire (*arrows*) extends from the left subclavian artery to the abdominal aorta.

B. Abnormal Air and Fluid Collections

Because air within the pleural cavity in supine and semirecumbent patients preferentially localizes to the anteromedial and subpulmonic recesses, radiographic manifestations of pneumothorax may be subtle. Early findings consist of asymmetric lucency over a hemidiaphragm or cardiac border and a deepened diaphragmatic sulcus (deep sulcus sign) (Fig. 9). Confirmation of pneumothorax is readily achieved by obtaining a radiograph with the patient in an upright or decubitus position with the involved side nondependent.

The radiographic findings of pneumomediastinum consist of lucent streaks that outline mediastinal structures, elevate the mediastinal pleura, and often extend into the neck and chest wall (subcutaneous emphysema) (Fig. 10A). Mediastinal gas situated along the superior margin of

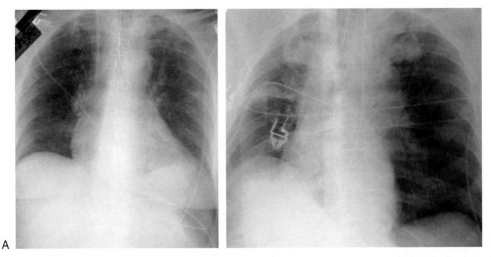

FIG. 9. Position and radiographic appearance of pneumothorax in supine patients. **A:** Asymmetric lucency over the left hemidiaphragm with deepened sulcus (deep sulcus sign) indicates the presence of left pneumothorax. **B:** Asymmetric lucency over the left hemidiaphragm associated with a mediastinal shift to the right indicates the presence of tension pneumothorax.

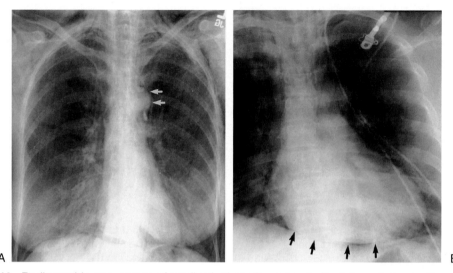

A   B

FIG. 10. Radiographic appearance of mediastinal emphysema. **A:** Radiolucent streaks throughout the mediastinum dissect into neck, chest wall, and retroperitoneum. Elevation of mediastinal pleura at the level of the aortic arch (*arrows*) clearly distinguishes between pneumomediastinum and pneumopericardium. **B:** Mediastinal gas creates a radiolucent line interposed between the heart and diaphragm (*arrows*) (continuous diaphragm sign).

the diaphragm creates a radiolucent line interposed between the heart and diaphragm (continuous diaphragm sign) (Fig. 10B).

Pleural effusions layer posteriorly in supine ICU patients. The characteristic radiographic manifestation of a unilateral pleural effusion is an asymmetric, diffuse, homogeneous opacity that increases in density in a cephalocaudad direction; lack of associated air bronchograms or obscuration of parenchymal vessels confirms that the increased opacity is extraparenchymal in location (silhouette sign).

C. Lung Parenchymal Diseases

The only direct radiographic sign of atelectasis is displacement of interlobar fissures (Fig. 11); all other commonly associated findings including increased density with air bronchograms and shift of hilar, mediastinal, and diaphragmatic structures may be caused by other processes such as infection and prior surgery, respectively. Transient, linear or bandlike opacities are characteristic of subsegmental atelectasis.

Radiographic distribution of parenchymal

consolidation in the earliest stage of ARDS reflects the type of inciting lung injury. A regional distribution is characteristic of focal processes such as aspiration (Fig. 12A) or pulmonary contusion as contrasted to a diffuse distribution resulting from global insults such as sepsis. In later

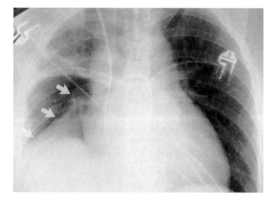

FIG. 11. Right lower lobe atelectasis in a 30-year-old man. Portable radiograph shows inferior displacement of the right major fissure (*arrows*) indicative of right lower lobe atelectasis. Associated indirect findings include mediastinal shift to right and elevation of right hemidiaphragm.

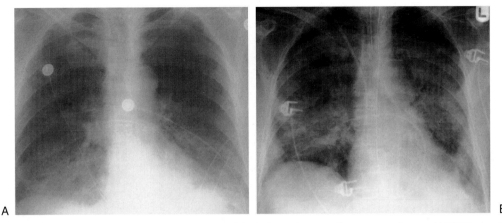

A   B

FIG. 12. Evolution of radiographic findings of acute respiratory distress syndrome (ARDS) due to aspiration in a 70-year-old man. **A:** In the early stage of ARDS, consolidation is present in a characteristic bibasilar, dependent distribution. **B:** Portable radiograph obtained 4 days after **(A)** shows a diffuse, bilateral, consolidative pattern indistinguishable in appearance from other causes of ARDS.

stages of ARDS, a diffuse, bilateral, consolidative pattern is characteristic (Fig. 12B); although every region of the lung is usually involved, the severity of consolidation is not uniform and some areas may be completely spared. CT and postmortem studies have demonstrated that consolidation in ARDS is often patchy and regional with a marked gravitational dependence even when distribution appears uniform on radiographs (Fig. 13).

Although new or changing opacities are the typical radiographic manifestations of pneumonia, these findings are neither sensitive nor specific for diagnosis of pulmonary infection in patients with preexisting ARDS. Rapid cavitation of a parenchymal abnormality is suggestive of a necrotizing VAP; however, no clinical or radiographic criteria have been found to reliably discriminate between ventilated patients with and without pneumonia.

V. SENSITIVITY AND SPECIFICITY

Few data are available regarding the sensitivity and specificity of portable radiographs and diagnosis of VAP or ARDS; based on the results of one study (5) of 40 patients, diagnostic accuracy (as defined by the area under receiver operating characteristic curve) of portable chest radiographs for VAP and ARDS was 0.52 and 0.84, respectively.

VI. DIFFERENTIAL DIAGNOSIS

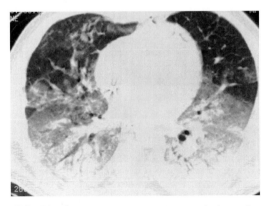

FIG. 13. Autopsy-proven acute respiratory distress syndrome associated with pneumonia in a 34-year-old man. Computed tomography scan obtained with 1-mm collimation shows bilateral, patchy consolidation predominating in dependent, posterior lower lobes.

Extraluminal gas in the mediastinum may represent either pneumomediastinum or pneumopericardium. In contrast to pneumomediastinum, pneumopericardium is an uncommon complication in ICU patients, usually only seen

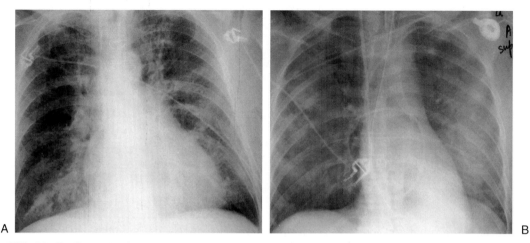

FIG. 14. Radiographic features of hydrostatic and increased-permeability pulmonary edema. **A:** Hydrostatic pulmonary edema is characterized by bilateral and symmetric distribution, multiple septal lines, peribronchial cuffing, and enlarged heart size. **B:** Increased-permeability edema is characterized by a diffuse, bilateral, consolidative pattern with prominent air bronchograms.

in association with recent cardiac surgery. The distribution of gas in pneumopericardium is limited to the confines of the pericardial sac, which extends superiorly to the level of the azygous vein, distal ascending aorta not including the aortic arch, and main pulmonary artery.

Differentiation between hydrostatic (cardiogenic, overhydration, and renal failure) and increased-permeability (injury) types of pulmonary edema may be difficult both clinically and radiographically; in some patients, both types may coexist. In general, the useful distinguishing radiographic features of hydrostatic edema are diffuse, symmetric distribution, septal lines, peribronchial cuffing, pleural effusion, and increased heart size and vascular pedicle width (Fig. 14A); in contrast, the characteristic radiographic pattern of increased-permeability edema is diffuse, patchy consolidation associated with prominent air bronchograms (Fig. 14B).

VII. PITFALLS

Difficulty in accurate radiographic diagnosis of VAP arises because parenchymal opacification, the hallmark of pneumonia, is a nonspecific finding that may be caused by noninfectious disorders such as atelectasis, bland aspiration, pulmonary embolism, atypical cardiogenic edema, and asymmetric ARDS. Conversely, the diffuse parenchymal abnormalities associated with ARDS often conceal superimposed infection. Reliable diagnosis of VAP often requires an invasive procedure such as bronchoscopy with sampling of secretions from the lower respiratory tract.

VIII. REFERENCES

1. Janower ML, Jennas-Nocera Z, Mukai J. Utility and efficacy of portable chest radiographs. *AJR Am J Radiol* 1984;142:265–267.
2. Henschke CI, Pasternack GS, Schroeder S, Hart KK, Herman PG. Bedside chest radiography: diagnostic efficacy. *Radiology* 1983;149:23–26.
3. Bekemeyer WB, Crapo RO, Calhoon S, Cannon CY, Clayton PD. Efficacy of chest radiography in a respiratory intensive care unit—a prospective study. *Chest* 1985;88:691–696.
4. Bernard GR, Artigas A, Brigham KL, et al. The American European Consensus Conference on ARDS—definitions, mechanisms, relevant outcomes, and clinical trial coordination. *Am J Respir Crit Care Med* 1994;149:818–824.
5. Winer-Muram HT, Rubin SA, Ellis JV, et al. Pneumonia and ARDS in patients receiving mechanical ventilation: diagnostic accuracy of chest radiography. *Radiology* 1993;188:479–485.

10

Blunt Abdominal Trauma

R. Brooke Jeffrey, Jr.

I. CLINICAL OVERVIEW

Computed tomography (CT) has had a major impact on the management of patients with blunt abdominal trauma. Prior to CT, peritoneal lavage to detect hemoperitoneum was the mainstay of diagnosis. Nonoperative management was often not possible because of the clinical inability to diagnose visceral injuries confidently. Many patients with relatively minor intraperitoneal injuries had a positive peritoneal lavage and as a result were subjected to a nontherapeutic laparotomy. Routine use of CT in hemodynamically stable patients with blunt abdominal trauma has substantially reduced the number of nontherapeutic laparotomies. Perhaps even more significantly, however, a large percentage of hepatic, mesenteric, and renal injuries can now be treated nonoperatively.

The development of helical (spiral) CT has improved parenchymal contrast enhancement for abdominal CT. The diagnosis of active arterial extravasation is much more readily apparent due to the improved vascular opacification that can be achieved with faster helical scanners. The CT diagnosis of active arterial extravasation frequently requires prompt intervention either with surgery or angiographic embolization. Significant blood loss results from nonoperative management in these patients.

II. IMAGING STRATEGY

At most trauma centers in the United States, CT is the primary imaging modality to evaluate hemodynamically stable patients with significant blunt abdominal trauma. There has been, however, an increasing interest in the role of sonography in the evaluation of blunt abdominal trauma both in Europe and North America. In most reports, the primary focus has been on the sonographic detection of the free intraperitoneal fluid presumed to be hemoperitoneum. Compared with CT, sonography has several important limitations in evaluating patients with blunt trauma. First, even when sonography detects free intraperitoneal fluid, CT will still be required to diagnose and stage the parenchymal injury that caused the hemoperitoneum. If surgery is performed purely on the basis of a positive sonogram (as with peritoneal lavage), a high incidence of nontherapeutic laparotomy will result. Secondly, sonography is relatively poor at detecting visceral lacerations or free intraperitoneal gas from a bowel perforation. Thirdly, a significant number of patients have visceral injuries without detectable hemoperitoneum that could potentially go undiagnosed with sonography. In a study of 772 patients who had sustained blunt abdominal trauma, Chiu noted that 29% of abdominal injuries had no associated hemoperitoneum; four patients in this series with splenic injury required laparotomy despite an initial negative sonogram. Fourthly, sonography cannot reliably detect retroperitoneal injuries. Therefore, lesions carrying a high morbidity, such as lacerations to the pancreas, duodenum, kidney, and retroperitoneal colon, will be missed by a ''negative'' sonogram for intraperitoneal fluid. Finally, bony injuries such as vertebral and pelvic fractures can be readily detected by CT but will be routinely missed by sonography. Sonography may prove to be useful to evaluate unstable patients who cannot undergo CT.

III. TECHNIQUE

Both oral and intravenous contrast should routinely be used for the CT evaluation of patients with blunt abdominal trauma. In conscious patients, oral contrast can be administered by mouth. Approximately 400 to 700 mL of water-soluble oral contrast is required to opacify the stomach, duodenum, and proximal small bowel. No attempt is made to opacify the distal small bowel due to the urgent time requirements to perform CT and the fact that distal small bowel and colonic injuries are relatively rare. A 1% solution of water-soluble contrast is generally administered via a nasogastric tube in unconscious patients. Before scanning, the nasogastric tube is withdrawn to the distal esophagus. At the end of the scan, the tube is reinserted into the stomach so the contents of the stomach can be aspirated.

Intravenous contrast is essential for diagnosis of visceral injuries and active arterial extravasation. Contrast is injected at a rate of 3 mL/s with a mechanical injector. A total of 150 mL of 60% iodinated contrast is administered. A single-portal venous phase acquisition is performed with a 60- to 70-second delay before image acquisition. For helical scans, a 7-mm collimation is used with a pitch of 1.5. The reconstruction interval is 7 mm. Scans are performed from just above the diaphragm to the symphysis pubis. It is important to view abdominal CT scans for trauma with multiple windows including lung windows to evaluate for pneumoperitoneum (Fig. 1), unsuspected pneumothorax, and bone windows to detect vertebral and pelvic fractures. Attenuation measurements are performed routinely for any abnormal fluid collections to distinguish blood (generally more than 25 Hounsfield units) (HU) from other serious fluid collection such as urine, bile, and chyle (HU less than 15).

IV. FINDINGS

A. Visceral Injuries

The most common visceral injuries are parenchymal lacerations and subcapsular hematomas (Fig. 2). Because these visceral injuries are avas-

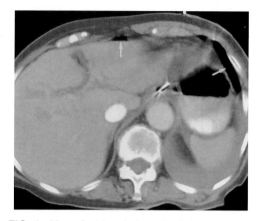

FIG. 1. Use of wide windows to detect pneumoperitoneum. Note free air seen anteriorly in the abdomen in this patient with bowel perforation following blunt abdominal trauma (*arrows*). The wide windows help to differentiate intraperitoneal fat from air.

cular, they will not significantly enhance after intravenous injection of contrast.

B. Attenuation Values for Blood

Free lysed hemoperitoneum is generally greater than 25 HU. If blood is mixed with bile (as with a hepatic laceration), the attenuation values may be somewhat less. Clotted blood contained within a visceral hematoma may approach 50 to 60 HU in attenuation. Foci of very high attenuation (isodense with major adjacent arterial structures adjacent to a visceral laceration) are diagnostic for active arterial extravasation (Fig. 3). The identification of active extravasation is of critical importance in patient management. In general, it implies that nonoperative management will result in significant blood loss and, therefore, either surgery or angiographic embolization is indicated. The site of active arterial extravasation often dictates clinical management. With intraperitoneal active bleeding, surgery is generally preferred as the mode of treatment. For extraperitoneal active arterial extravasation (such as from a lumbar artery distribution), angiographic embolization is often the most effective therapy (Fig. 4). Surgery for

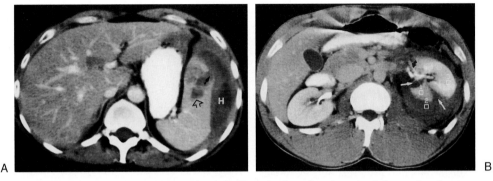

FIG. 2. Low-attenuating visceral lacerations. **A:** Note the low-density splenic laceration (*open arrow*) with interruption of the splenic capsule (*arrow*). A subcapsular hematoma (*H*) is seen flattening a lateral contour of the spleen. **B:** In another patient, note low attenuation of wedge-shaped left renal lacerations (*arrows*). Extravasation from the collecting system is also noted (*curved black arrow*).

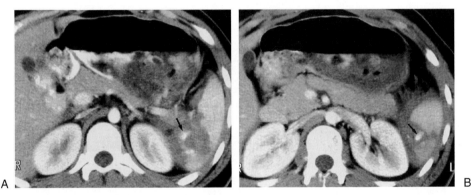

FIG. 3. Active arterial extravasation from splenic laceration. **A** and **B:** Note foci of high attenuation (*arrows*) within the low-density splenic laceration. At surgery, active arterial extravasation was noted from the lower pole of the spleen.

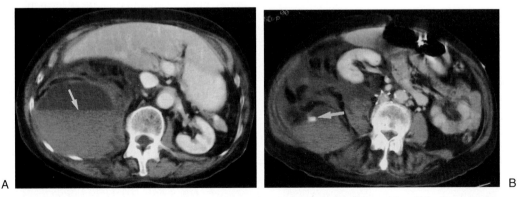

FIG. 4. Retroperitoneal active arterial extravasation from a lumbar artery bleed. **A:** Note the large retroperitoneal hematoma with hematocrit effect (*arrow*). **B:** A focus of active arterial extravasation (*arrow*) arises from a lacerated lumbar artery. Angiographic embolization of the lumbar artery was successful in controlling the hemorrhage.

lumbar artery extravasation is often hazardous and time consuming.

C. Injuries to the Gastrointestinal Tract

Intramural hematomas and lacerations to the gastrointestinal tract generally occur at sites of relative bowel fixation such as the duodenum and jejunum near the ligament of Treitz (Fig. 5). Seat belt injuries may be associated with injuries to the distal small bowel and retroperitoneal colon. Small bowel injuries to the proximal jejunum just beyond the ligament of Treitz are the most common small bowel lacerations. Because this portion of the gastrointestinal tract frequently does not contain gas, pneumoperitoneum is frequently not present with jejunal lacerations. Free intraperitoneal fluid representing luminal contents of the small bowel (HU less than 15) frequently locates between the reflections of the small bowel mesentery (the intraloop compartment). Water-density intraloop fluid may be the only sign of small bowel perforation in these patients (Fig. 6).

Intramural hematomas of the bowel may result in diffuse mural thickening. This is often best appreciated with oral contrast outlining the narrowed lumen. Extravasation of oral contrast is direct evidence of bowel perforation (Fig. 7). The extravasated contents may also be within an intraloop location or spread to other peritoneal spaces such as the paracolic gutters or subphrenic spaces. Pneumoperitoneum is often noted along the anterior abdominal wall in a supine patient (Fig. 8). In some patients, however, gas bubbles may be trapped by intraperitoneal ligaments such as gastrohepatic and gastroduodenal ligaments. In other patients small gas bubbles may be trapped within the interstices of the greater omentum and are seen adjacent to loops of small bowel or colon.

D. Useful Signs in CT of Trauma

1. The Sentinel Clot Sign

This sign refers to the fact that the higher the attenuation of blood, the closer the anatomic site of visceral injury. Free lysed blood in the peritoneal cavity typically has attenuation values of greater than 25 HU. Clotted blood may be on the order of 50 to 60 HU (Fig. 9). In subtle cases of trauma, an adjacent collection of blood (sentinel clot) may be the only sign of visceral trauma.

2. The Collapsed Cava Sign

Hypovolemia may result in diffuse flattening of the intra- and extrahepatic inferior vena cava. When this finding is present, it is important to alert the clinicians to the requirement for central venous pressure monitoring to adequately replace blood volume.

3. Shock Nephrograms

In patients who are hypotensive, delayed transit of contrast through the kidney is noted with absence of excretion if the blood pressure drops, typically below 60 to 70 mm Hg.

4. The Small Hypodense Spleen

In patients who have sustained hemorrhagic shock and then have been resuscitated, the spleen may be small and diffusely hypoattenuating due to intense vasoconstriction of the splenic

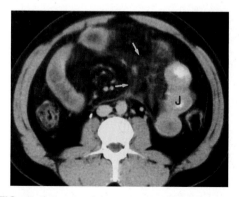

FIG. 5. Intramural hematoma of the jejunum. Note bowel thickening of the jejunum (*J*) with adjacent edema and hematoma in the small bowel mesentery (*arrows*).

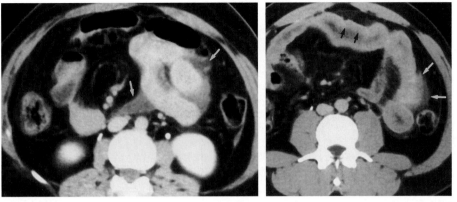

A   B

FIG. 6. The water-density intraloop fluid as the only sign of bowel perforation. **A:** Note triangular collections of intraloop fluid adjacent to the jejunum (*arrows*). Small bowel perforation was proven at surgery. Note the lack of pneumoperitoneum. **B:** In another patient, note the mural thickening of the jejunum (*black arrows*). Extravasated water-density fluid is seen adjacent to the bowel. Jejunal perforation was diagnosed at surgery.

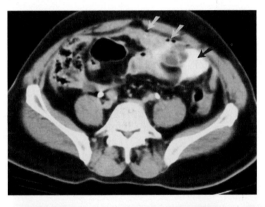

FIG. 7. Extravasation of oral contrast from bowel perforation. Note the triangular intraloop collection of high-density oral contrast (*black arrow*) adjacent to the jejunum. Ectopic gas bubbles are also seen in the peritoneal cavity anteriorly (*white arrows*).

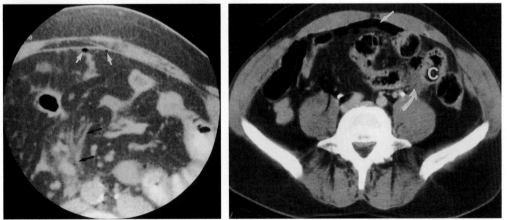

A   B

FIG. 8. Pneumoperitoneum from bowel rupture in two patients. **A:** Note the tiny gas bubbles of pneumoperitoneum along the intraabdominal wall (*white arrows*); a small mesenteric hematoma is noted within the mesentery (*black arrows*). **B:** In another patient, note the pneumoperitoneum along the anterior abdominal wall (*white arrow*). High-density hematoma (curved arrow) is seen adjacent to a thickened sigmoid colon (*C*). Colonic perforation was diagnosed at surgery.

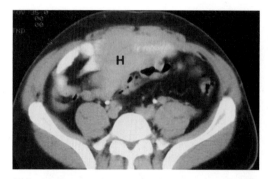

FIG. 9. Sentinel clot sign of mesenteric injury. Note the high-density hematoma (*H*) involving the distal small bowel and mesentery indicative of a mesenteric vascular injury.

artery (Fig. 10). This phenomenon will reverse after the patient stabilizes and no longer has circulating normetanephrines associated with hypotension and shock.

V. SENSITIVITY AND SPECIFICITY

General CT is highly sensitive and specific for visceral injuries. In a small percentage of patients, hemoperitoneum is noted without obvious visceral injury. In most of these instances, no surgery is required in these patients with presumed small mesenteric or hepatic lacerations that are of no clinical consequence. CT is more

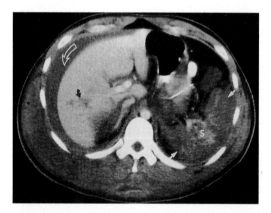

FIG. 10. Small hypodense spleen as a sign of shock. Note the low-attenuating spleen (*S*) of diminished size. Arrows indicate splenic contours. Hemoperitoneum (*curved white arrows*) is noted from a hepatic laceration (*curved black arrow*). At surgery, the spleen was normal.

reliable than plain films for the detection of subtle pneumothorax and subtle pneumoperitoneum.

VI. DIFFERENTIAL DIAGNOSIS

In the setting of blunt trauma, the differential diagnosis of visceral injuries is limited. In rare instances, underlying hepatic or renal neoplasms may be associated with acute intraperitoneal hemorrhage after minor trauma, which may be difficult to differentiate from underlying parenchymal lacerations. In general, the hepatic and renal tumors are more rounded and have more significant mass effect than parenchymal lacerations, which tend to be jagged and irregular.

VII. PITFALLS

A small percentage of pancreatic and gastrointestinal lesions may be impossible to diagnose with CT soon after injury. Pancreatic lacerations may be subtle, and the most obvious feature of injury to the pancreas on CT is the detection of peripancreatic fluid collection within the anterior pararenal space along Gerota's fascia. The changes of post-traumatic pancreatitis are often time dependent and may not be evident within the first few hours after visceral injury. A useful CT finding of pancreatic injuries is retroperitoneal fluid representing extravasation of pancreatic juice from the main pancreatic duct. In most patients, there is no clearly defined fat plane between the posterior margin of the pancreas and the splenic vein. Fluid collecting between the splenic vein and the pancreas strongly suggests pancreatic injury. Follow-up scans or endoscopic retrograde cannulation of the pancreatic duct may be useful in selected patients who are clinically at high risk for pancreatic injury.

At times, gastrointestinal injuries may produce subtle features such as tiny pneumoperitoneum or small intraloop fluid collections. Therefore, a dedicated search must be made using very wide windows, carefully looking for pneumoperitoneum and searching all intraperitoneal spaces for free intraabdominal fluid collections.

Splenic lacerations rarely may not be evident on the initial CT (Fig. 11). Repeat CT should be

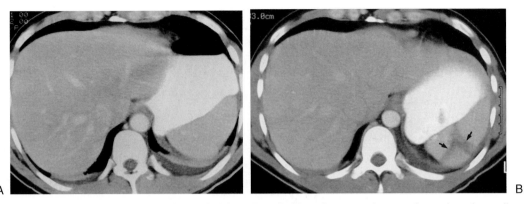

FIG. 11. Delayed visualization of splenic laceration. **A:** Note the normal-appearing spleen immediately after injury. **B:** Two days later, splenic lacerations are now clearly evident (*arrows*).

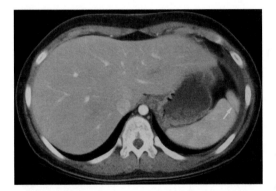

FIG. 12. Congenital splenic cleft mimicking laceration. Note the linear area along the inferior pole of the spleen consistent with a splenic cleft (*arrow*).

performed in any patient with delayed symptoms due to this potential pitfall. Splenic clefts are linear low-attenuation bands that may rarely mimic lacerations (Fig. 12). The absence of perisplenic blood is a useful observation. Infarcts of the spleen or kidney may at times mimic lacerations (Fig. 13). A capsular rim sign is diagnostic of an infarct. A cortical rim sign is a typical feature of a renal infarct not evident with trauma.

Foci of active arterial extravasation may at times mimic the attenuation of oral contrast. However, there is invariably a larger adjacent hematoma and an associated visceral laceration.

VIII. SUGGESTED READINGS

Chiu WC, Cushing BM, Rodriguez A, et al. Abdominal injuries without hemoperitoneum: a potential limitation of focused abdominal sonography for trauma. *J Trauma* 1197; 42(4):617–623.

Federle MP, Jeffrey RB Jr. Hemoperitoneum studied by computed tomography. *Radiology* 1983;148:187–192.

Jeffrey RB Jr, Cardoza JD, Olcott EW. Detection of active intraabdominal arterial hemorrhage: value of dynamic contrast-enhanced CT. *AJR Am J Radiol* 1991;158: 725–729.

Orwig D, Federle MP. Localized clotted blood as evidence of visceral trauma on CT: the sentinel clot sign. *AJR Am J Radiol* 1989;153:747–749.

Wing VW, Federle MP, Morris JA Jr, Jeffrey RB Jr, Bluth R. The clinical impact of CT for blunt abdominal trauma. *AJR Am J Radiol* 1985;145:1191–1194.

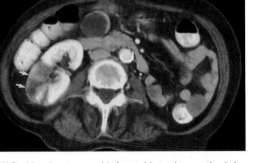

FIG. 13. Acute renal infarct. Note the cortical rim sign (*arrows*), which helps differentiate an infarct from a parenchymal laceration.

11

Right Upper Quadrant Pain

Rule Out Acute Cholecystitis

Philip W. Ralls

I. CLINICAL OVERVIEW

Patients with acute cholecystitis almost always present with constant right upper quadrant pain (biliary colic), fever, and leukocytosis. Despite classic signs and symptoms, the clinical diagnosis of acute cholecystitis is often challenging and may be incorrect in more than one-third of patients. Clearly, confirmation of the diagnosis is needed before surgery can be performed.

In the United States alone it is estimated that more than 20 million individuals have gallstones. Gallstone disease is the most common cause of hospitalization in the United States. Acute cholecystitis is the most severe form of gallbladder disease. A gallstone obstructing the cystic duct causes approximately 90% to 95% of acute cholecystitis cases. The remaining cases are unrelated to gallstones (acute acalculous cholecystitis) and are usually ischemic in origin. Acalculous cholecystitis is unusual as a presenting condition. It most often occurs as a complication of other diseases in critically ill or immunocompromised patients. Patients with acute cholecystitis do best with early cholecystectomy, performed within 24 to 72 hours of presentation. They have shorter hospitalizations and fewer complications, such as pericholecystic abscess (Fig. 1) or gallbladder perforation (Fig. 2), than patients managed conservatively.

Sonography provides an accurate, quick diagnosis of acute cholecystitis. Technetium 99m image display and analysis (IDA) cholescintig-raphy can also effectively screen patients with suspected acute cholecystitis. Because both are useful, the test chosen for screening depends on local practice conditions.

II. IMAGING STRATEGY

Sonography and cholescintigraphy are comparatively accurate, at about the 90% level in prospective trials. Positive sonography for acute cholecystitis is more reliable than cholescintig-raphy—positive sonographic findings strongly indicate the presence of acute cholecystitis. False-positive results are rare with sonography and common with cholescintigraphy. On the other hand, a negative cholescintigram (radionuclide filling of the gallbladder) is more reliable than a negative sonogram in ruling out acute cholecystitis. Cholescintigraphy can be used effectively as a screening tool for patients with suspected acute cholecystitis. Sonography and cholescintigraphy are complementary tests. Each can be used to clarify equivocal results when the other is used first.

We prefer sonography for evaluating patients with suspected acute cholecystitis. Surgeons like the reliability of sonography to diagnose gallstones. Sonography has a high predictive value (positive predictive value, PPV, about 99%) for patients who need cholecystectomy. Unlike scintigraphy, sonography is not "organ specific." When the gallbladder is normal, sonography can be used to rapidly survey the remainder of the abdomen to search for an alternative cause

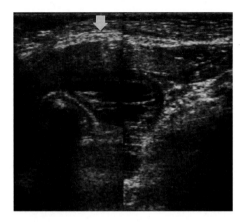

FIG. 1. Acute cholecystitis with pericholecystic abscess. This transverse composite sonogram delineates stones in the gallbladder and a large septated pericholecystic abscess. Note the echogenic inflammation in the anterior abdominal wall (*arrow*).

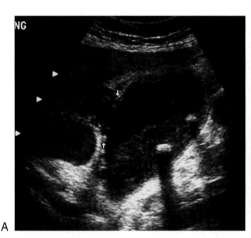

A

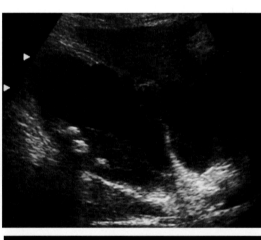

B

FIG. 2. Pericholecystic abscess with perforation. The longitudinal sonogram **(A)** shows sludge in the gallbladder, multiple gallstones, and a gallbladder wall perforation (*tiny arrows*). The echogenic submucosa is interrupted at the level of the arrows, and free perforation into the pericholecystic region is noted. A transverse sonogram **(B)** reveals the greater extent of the pericholecystic abscess. A computed tomography scan **(C)** also shows the pericholecystic collection, although it does not show the wall disruption as clearly as the sonogram does. Perforation of the gallbladder is a prerequisite to a pericholecystic abscess. Usually interruption of the submucosa is the most reliable sign of gallbladder perforation. In our experience, gall-bladder wall perforation cannot be definitively demonstrated in all patients with pericholecystic abscess.

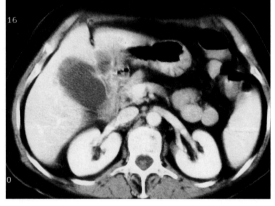

C

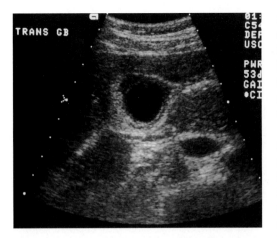

FIG. 3. Acute acalculous cholecystitis. This transverse sonogram of the gallbladder shows thickening of the gallbladder wall, the only finding in this patient with acute cholecystitis. Imaging diagnosis of acalculous cholecystitis is difficult. Increasing gallbladder wall thickening on serial studies or the detection of inflammation contiguous to the gallbladder by computed tomography or sonography can facilitate the diagnosis.

of the patient's right upper quadrant pain. It is superior to cholescintigraphy in its ability to detect and characterize complications of acute cholecystitis. Sonography can also guide diagnostic aspiration and biopsy and therapeutic percutaneous cholecystostomy or abscess drainage, when needed.

Computed tomography (CT) is not a primary means of assessing patients with calculous acute cholecystitis, but CT may discover it when performed in a patient with abdominal pain. CT is less sensitive than sonography in detecting gallstones (70% versus 95% for sonography), but it does have an advantage in demonstrating inflammation, mainly by showing abnormal pericholecystic fat. Use of CT is more important in patients with suspected acute acalculous cholecystitis.

A. Acute Acalculous Cholecystitis

Acute acalculous cholecystitis is often extremely difficult to diagnose by imaging or clinical criteria (Figs. 3, 4, and 5; Color Plates 1 and 2). Even the use of percutaneous gallbladder

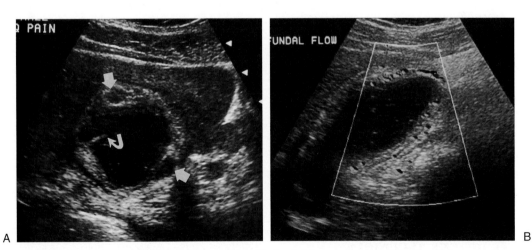

A   B

FIG. 4. Gangrenous acalculous cholecystitis with fundal flow on power Doppler. This patient presented with right upper quadrant pain, fever, and a normal white cell count. Gray-scale imaging **(A)** revealed a markedly abnormal gallbladder with wall thickening, sludge, mural irregularities, intramural abscesses (*arrows*) and an intraluminal membrane (*curved arrow*). Prominent fundal flow was present on both power **(B)** and color Doppler. Although more common in acute cholecystitis, normal fundal flow is now often seen because of the improved sensitivity of newer Doppler systems. (See also Color Plate 1.)

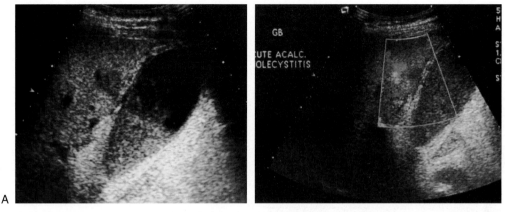

FIG. 5. Acute acalculous cholecystitis with increased mural flow. A longitudinal gray-scale sonogram **(A)** shows sludge in the gallbladder and a thickened, striated gallbladder wall. No gallstones were discovered. **B:** The color Doppler sonogram shows flow in the cystic artery throughout the wall. These findings, in the correct clinical setting, suggest acute acalculous cholecystitis. (See also Color Plate 2.)

aspiration for culture is unreliable. Acalculous cholecystitis is often detected only because of its complications. Many have advocated empiric percutaneous gallbladder drainage when acute acalculous cholecystitis is suspected. We feel this approach is prudent because acute acalculous cholecystitis often cannot be identified at an early stage.

Several strategies may prove useful in facilitating a more accurate image diagnosis of acute acalculous cholecystitis. Pericholecystic abnormalities detected on CT scans are often more useful than screening sonograms or cholescintigraphy (Figs. 6 and 7). Sequential CT or ultrasound examination may show progressive thickening of the gallbladder wall. Color Doppler sonography may reveal hyperemia in the gallbladder wall (see Figs. 4 and 5), although this is an imperfect diagnostic sign. Perhaps future developments in imaging will eventually solve this challenging problem.

III. TECHNIQUE

A. Sonography

Sonography is best performed with 3- to 5-MHz curved linear or sector transducers. Many modern systems can image the gallbladder comfortably at 7 MHz. When preliminary scanning is negative, scans with higher frequency can show small or difficult-to-image stones not visible with lower frequency transducers (Fig. 8). Tissue harmonic imaging may be useful to further clarify gallbladder pathology. Gallstones are most difficult to detect when they are impacted in the cystic duct, a common location in patients with acute cholecystitis. Some stones in the cystic duct will inevitably be missed. To minimize this, attempt to visualize the entrance of the cystic duct into the extrahepatic common duct when stones have not already been detected. Using transverse scans, follow the common hepatic duct caudally from the porta hepatis until the cystic duct is seen entering the common duct. If this fails, trace the cystic duct from the gallbladder neck into the common duct. The junction of the cystic and extrahepatic ducts will not always be visualized, but the attempt will minimize the number of cystic duct stones that are missed (Fig. 9). Even when sonography does not detect gallstones, acute cholecystitis is not totally excluded. Acute calculous cholecystitis caused by an undetected cystic duct stone or acute acalculous cholecystitis may be present. Cholescintigraphy should be performed when clinical suspicion persists in such patients.

Gallbladder wall thickness should be measured perpendicular to the ventral wall on long

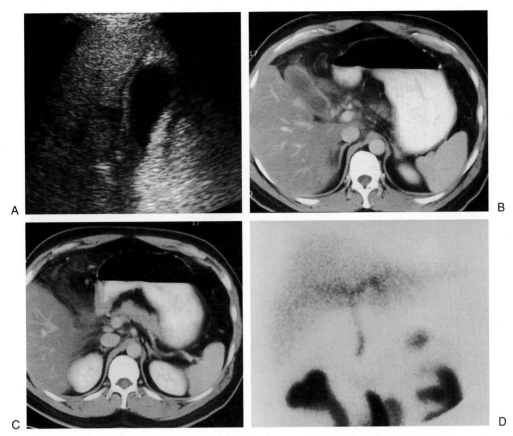

FIG. 6. Acute acalculous cholecystitis. A sonogram of the gallbladder **(A)** reveals gallbladder wall thickening and decreased pericholecystic echogenicity most likely related to edema from inflammation. No stones are identified. The computed tomography (CT) scan performed the same day shows an irregular, thick-walled gallbladder with pericholecystic inflammation seen as increased density within the fat **(B** and **C)**. A technetium 99m image display and analysis cholescintigram after morphine injection shows no filling of the gallbladder **(D)**, a positive study. Acute acalculous cholecystitis may be difficult to diagnose. Visualization of pericholecystic inflammation on CT is one of the better signs allowing diagnosis of this condition.

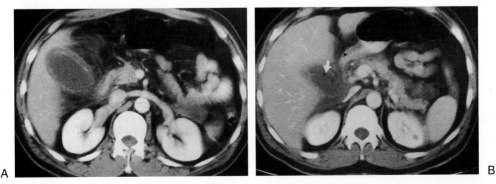

FIG. 7. Acute acalculous cholecystitis. This diabetic man presented with severe right upper quadrant pain. A computed tomography scan **(A)** through the mid gallbladder reveals thickening of the gallbladder wall with some higher attenuation areas in the wall, probably from mural hemorrhage. The most striking abnormality is the pericholecystic inflammation in the fat adjacent to the gallbladder. A scan at a more cephalic level **(B)** reveals fine gas bubbles within the gallbladder wall (*arrow*). Emphysematous cholecystitis is most common in diabetics. This primary presentation of acute acalculous cholecystitis is unusual because most patients with emphysematous cholecystitis have gallstones.

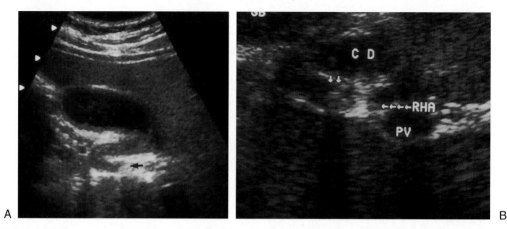

FIG. 8. Cystic duct stones seen only with 7-MHz scanning. Most missed gallstones are present in the cystic duct. High-frequency scanning and careful technique are necessary to visualize these stones. This stone was completely invisible with 3- and 5-MHz transducers. A small cystic duct stone (*tiny arrow*) is seen shadowing in the unmagnified sonogram **(A)**. The magnified sonogram **(B)** shows the relationship of the cystic duct stone (*arrows pointing down*) to the common duct (*CD*). Careful technique coupled with high-frequency scanning allowed visualization of this stone. RHA, right hepatic artery; PV, main portal vein.

axis scans, in the mid gallbladder. Greater than 3 mm is considered abnormal. The sonographic Murphy sign should be recorded. Misconceptions regarding the sonographic Murphy sign are common. A positive sonographic Murphy sign consists of maximum reproducible tenderness over the sonographically localized gallbladder. *When tenderness is not reproducibly maximal over the gallbladder, the sonographic Murphy sign is negative.* If there is any question whether the sonographic Murphy sign is positive, it is then considered negative. *An "equivocal" sonographic Murphy sign is a negative sonography Murphy sign.*

B. Biliary Scintigraphy

Optimally, the patient should be fasting for 4 to 6 hours before the examination. A dose of 3 to 5 mCi of ^{99m}Tc IDA is injected intravenously. A large field-of-view camera is set up for ^{99m}Tc imaging with the liver in the right upper portion

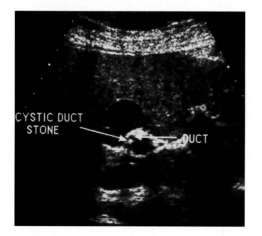

FIG. 9. Tiny cystic duct stone. No gallstones were detected in the gallbladder in this patient with suspected cholelithiasis. A careful evaluation of the cystic duct region is appropriate because most gallbladder stones that are missed are in the cystic duct. Ideally, the cystic duct should be followed to its entrance into the extrahepatic bile duct. This patient has a tiny cystic duct stone seen in the distal cystic duct just before it enters the extrahepatic duct (*DUCT*). Small stones in the cystic duct are easily missed. On occasion, even large stones in the cystic duct may be missed sonographically.

of the field of view. Images of 500,000 to 750,000 counts are obtained every 5 minutes for the first 30 minutes, then every 10 minutes for the next 30 minutes. If there is no visualization of the gallbladder at 1 hour, morphine is given (0.04 mg/kg intravenously) to cause spasm of the sphincter of Oddi, forcing radionuclide into the gallbladder if the cystic duct is open. Image for 20 to 60 minutes after morphine injection.

IV. RADIOGRAPHIC FINDINGS

A. Sonography

Sonographic detection of gallstones alone is not sufficient to definitively diagnose acute cholecystitis. Although finding gallstones in patients with suspected acute cholecystitis strongly suggests that diagnosis, it is not unusual to detect incidental gallstones that are not responsible for the patient's problem. Because of this, supporting secondary sonographic signs of acute cholecystitis have been developed and evaluated. The two signs most useful in patients with suspected acute cholecystitis are a positive sonographic Murphy sign and gallbladder wall thickening (Figs. 8 and 10). In a patient with suspected acute cholecystitis, the presence of either of these signs plus gallstones yields a PPV of more than 99% for patients whose pain is cured by cholecystectomy. The PPV for pathologically correlated acute cholecystitis is 92% to 95%. The others have chronic cholecystitis pathologically.

It is important to remember that secondary supporting signs should be used *only in those patients with suspected acute cholecystitis*. Finding gallstones and either a thickened gallbladder wall or gallstones and a positive sonographic

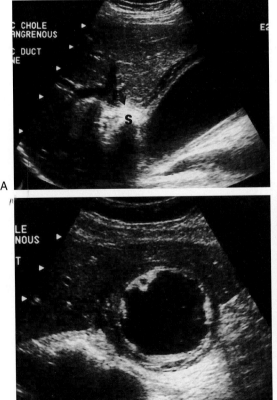

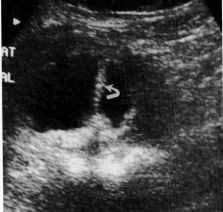

FIG. 10. Gangrenous acute cholecystitis. This case displays the classic findings of gangrenous acute cholecystitis. A cystic duct stone (*S*) is present. Note the increased echogenicity fat around the neck and cystic duct of the gallbladder (*arrow*). This echogenic fat is indicative of inflammation. Gallbladder wall striations are present. Transverse images (**B** and **C**) show sloughing of the mucosa in addition to the wall striations. An intraluminal membrane (*curved arrow*) is seen near the gallbladder fundus.

A

B

C

Murphy sign in a patient with fever, leukocytosis, and right upper quadrant pain strongly suggests the diagnosis of acute cholecystitis. It is this group of patients in whom surgeons wish to perform early cholecystectomy to forestall complications. Outpatients with chronic cholecystitis do not need early cholecystectomy. Elective cholecystectomy is appropriate. Although patients with chronic cholecystitis sometimes have thick gallbladder walls or even a positive Murphy sign, the information does not affect management. The presence of gallstones is the most useful information.

Other signs of acute cholecystitis are less useful. Color flow in the gallbladder fundus is now seen in many normal patients because of improved system Doppler sensitivity (see Figs. 4 and 5). Inflamed omental and pericholecystic fat (Figs. 10 and 11) is a useful finding but is not identified commonly. Definitive signs of severe acute cholecystitis such as mural gas (emphysematous cholecystitis) (Figs. 7 and 12) and pericholecystic abscess (see Figs. 1 and 2) are, fortunately, uncommon. Hyperemia of the inflamed omental fat may be demonstrated with color Doppler imaging (Fig. 13 and Color Plate 3).

1. Gangrenous Cholecystitis

Although gangrenous cholecystitis clearly has a higher rate of complications, diagnosing gangrenous acute cholecystitis should have little or no impact on patient outcome in most situations. If standard therapy (early cholecystectomy) is used, patient management is usually unaffected. On the other hand, diagnosing gangrenous cholecystitis may be useful if it prompts earlier surgery or if it aids in the decision to perform open rather than laparoscopic cholecystectomy.

A high percentage of patients with gangrenous acute cholecystitis do not have a positive sonographic Murphy sign, although the vast majority of these patients have marked gallbladder wall thickening and other mural abnormalities. Thus, most patients with acute cholecystitis with negative sonographic Murphy signs have abnormal gallbladder walls. Most patients with acute cholecystitis with normal gallbladder walls have positive sonographic Murphy signs.

Sonographic features that in the correct clinical situation suggest gangrenous cholecystitis include gallbladder wall striations (Figs. 4, 10, and 14), pericholecystic abscess (see Figs. 1 and 2), intraluminal membranes (due to sloughed

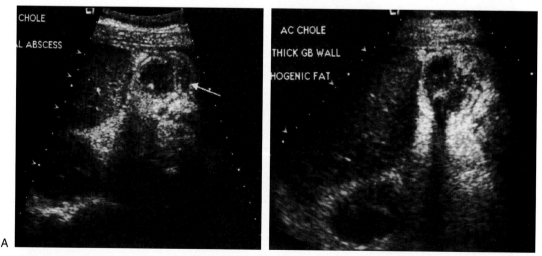

A   B

FIG. 11. Acute cholecystitis with echogenic fat and a mural abscess. The longitudinal sonogram **(A)** in this patient with gangrenous acute cholecystitis has a focal sonolucent abscess (*arrow*) in the gallbladder wall. Markedly echogenic fat adjacent to the gallbladder indicates pericholecystic inflammation **(B)**.

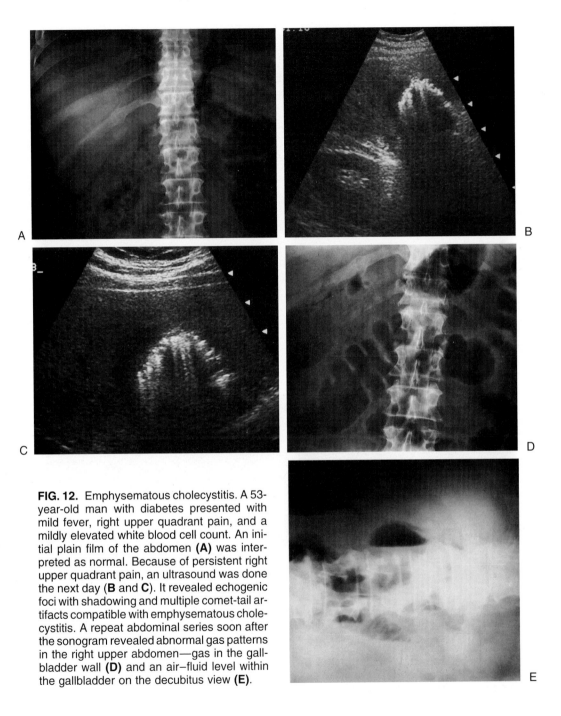

FIG. 12. Emphysematous cholecystitis. A 53-year-old man with diabetes presented with mild fever, right upper quadrant pain, and a mildly elevated white blood cell count. An initial plain film of the abdomen (**A**) was interpreted as normal. Because of persistent right upper quadrant pain, an ultrasound was done the next day (**B** and **C**). It revealed echogenic foci with shadowing and multiple comet-tail artifacts compatible with emphysematous cholecystitis. A repeat abdominal series soon after the sonogram revealed abnormal gas patterns in the right upper abdomen—gas in the gallbladder wall (**D**) and an air–fluid level within the gallbladder on the decubitus view (**E**).

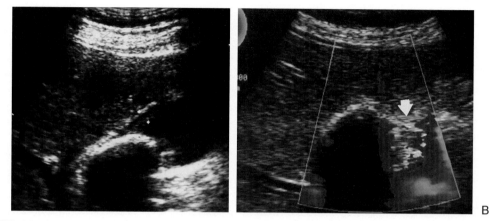

A   B

FIG. 13. Acute cholecystitis with increased flow in inflamed fat. The longitudinal sonogram **(A)** shows a gallstone and gallbladder wall thickening. The transverse power Doppler sonogram **(B)** shows increased flow in the echogenic, inflamed fat (*arrow*) medial to the gallbladder. Echogenic fat with increased flow supports the diagnosis of acute cholecystitis. (See also Color Plate 3.)

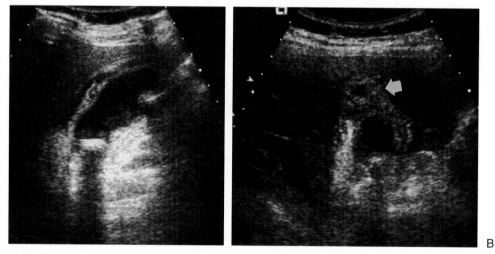

A   B

FIG. 14. Gangrenous acute calculous cholecystitis. A longitudinal sonogram **(A)** shows gallstones and a thickened gallbladder wall with mural striations. These findings are nearly diagnostic of gangrenous acute cholecystitis in a patient with right upper quadrant pain, fever, and an elevated white blood cell count. A transverse sonogram **(B)** shows similar findings, but the tangential nature of the scan plane accentuates the thickness of the edematous inflamed gallbladder wall (*arrow*). Thickened gallbladder walls are often misdiagnosed as pericholecystic abscesses.

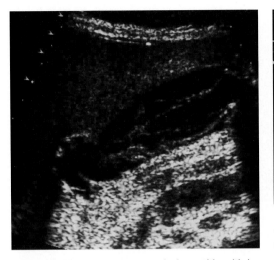

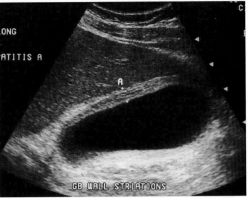

FIG. 17. Gallbladder wall thickening with striations from hepatitis A. This longitudinal image of the gallbladder shows a gallbladder wall that measures 7 mm. Note the linear striations seen more clearly in the ventral wall. Gallbladder wall thickening and gallbladder striations are nonspecific findings. Although they represent evidence for gangrenous cholecystitis in the correct clinical setting, other conditions have similar findings. Hepatitis A, hypoalbuminemia coupled with portal hypertension in cirrhosis, and human immunodeficiency virus cholangiopathy, among others, can cause similar findings in the absence of gangrenous cholecystitis.

FIG. 15. Gangrenous acute cholecystitis with intraluminal membrane. A longitudinal sonogram shows extensive delamination of the necrotic gallbladder mucosa in this patient with gangrenous cholecystitis. Intraluminal membranes are an unusual but virtually definitive sign for gangrenous acute cholecystitis. On occasion, sludge can mimic intraluminal membranes. Gallstones were present but not seen on this particular image.

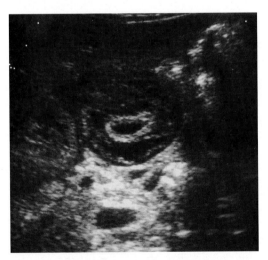

FIG. 16. Gallbladder wall thickening and wall striations from hepatitis A. This patient presented with fever and right upper quadrant pain. No stones were seen, but there was a markedly thickened gallbladder wall (greater than 1 cm). In addition, prominent gallbladder wall striations (mural edema) are present. This patient had hepatitis A, a common cause of gallbladder wall thickening with striations.

mucosa) (Figs. 10 and 15, and gas in the gallbladder wall (emphysematous cholecystitis) (see Figs. 7 and 12). Unfortunately, most mural abnormalities—wall thickening, gallbladder wall striations (Figs. 16 and 17), and intraluminal membranes (Fig. 18)—may be found in patients who do not have acute cholecystitis or even intrinsic gallbladder disease. Acute hepatitis (especially hepatitis A), hypoalbuminemia with portal hypertension, human immunodeficiency virus cholangiopathy, and occasionally congestive heart failure or renal failure may all cause wall thickening with striations (see Figs. 16 and 17).

B. Biliary Scintigraphy

In a normal cholecystogram, the gallbladder fills, excluding cystic duct obstruction and, thus, acute cholecystitis. Nonvisualization of the gallbladder at 1 hour is a positive study for acute cholecystitis (see Fig. 6), provided that the liver

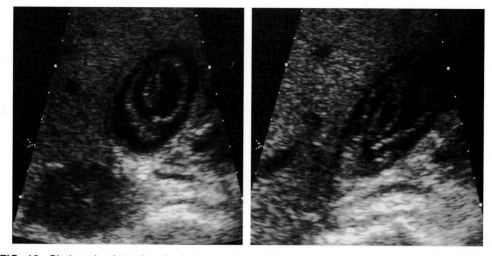

A   B

FIG. 18. Sludge simulates intraluminal membrane. The transverse **(A)** and longitudinal **(B)** sonograms of the gallbladder in this patient with fever and right upper quadrant pain reveal multiple linear structures that have the appearance of intraluminal membranes. This is not gangrenous cholecystitis but rather an unusual appearance of sludge within the gallbladder.

and bile ducts are normal and the radionuclide passes into the bowel. Increased flow in the gallbladder fossa and a rim sign on early flow images are additional signs of acute cholecystitis. Delayed filling indicates chronic cholecystitis. This is facilitated by morphine administration.

V. SENSITIVITY AND SPECIFICITY

Accuracy rates for sonography and cholescintigraphy in calculous acute cholecystitis are comparable, at about the 90% level. In a patient with suspected acute cholecystitis, the presence of gallstones on sonography plus either a positive sonographic Murphy sign or gallbladder wall thickening yields a PPV of more than 99% for patients whose pain is cured by cholecystectomy. Diagnosing acalculous cholecystitis is problematic. Accuracy ranges from 50% to 70% for both cholescintigraphy and sonography.

VI. DIFFERENTIAL DIAGNOSIS

A. Acute Pancreatitis

Acute pancreatitis may present with symptoms similar to those of acute cholecystitis. Because gallstones are a frequent cause of pancreatitis, the diagnosis may be problematic. Generally, the sonographic Murphy sign is negative, but pancreatitis is one of the more common causes of a false-positive sonographic Murphy sign. When the pancreas or peripancreatic regions are abnormal, or when tenderness is maximal over the pancreas, the diagnosis is clear. Hyperamylasemia and, especially, elevated serum lipase levels are useful laboratory findings.

B. Perforated Duodenal Ulcer

Perforated duodenal ulcer usually causes much more severe and acute pain than does acute cholecystitis. Collapse and shock often occur. Free intraperitoneal air, usually discovered on plain radiographs, is the radiographic hallmark, although it is not universally present. Sonography and especially CT may also reveal free intraperitoneal air. These findings generally suffice to distinguish perforated duodenal ulcer from acute cholecystitis. When the ulcer perforation is less massive, the symptoms may be less severe. Sonography does not reveal signs of acute cholecystitis in this circumstance.

C. Right Upper Quadrant Abscess

Subhepatic, subphrenic, and liver abscess may all simulate acute cholecystitis clinically. Detection of the abscess in the absence of findings for acute cholecystitis leads to a correct diagnosis.

D. Right-sided Pyelonephritis

Right-sided pyelonephritis may cause clinical confusion with acute cholecystitis. Even when the kidney is normal sonographically (as it is in most patients), focal renal tenderness may suggest the diagnosis. Again, absence of findings for acute cholecystitis leads to a correct diagnosis.

VII. PITFALLS

False-negative sonograms are the biggest problem in the sonographic diagnosis of acute cholecystitis. Although rare, acute cholecystitis can be missed when cystic duct stones are not detected, especially when the sonographic Murphy sign is negative and the gallbladder wall is normal. Acalculous cholecystitis is also a problematic diagnosis. False-positive results for acute calculous cholecystitis are rare if the secondary signs of wall thickening and positive sonographic results are used appropriately. Coincidental gallstones occasionally cause difficulties, especially in pancreatitis. This is not a significant clinical outcome problem, however, because all patients with pancreatitis with gallstones require cholecystectomy.

False-positive cholescintigrams (nonfilling of the gallbladder when acute cholecystitis is not present) are a problem. Although not frequent when morphine is given as part of the examination, false-positive results may lead to unnecessary surgery, an untoward outcome.

VIII. SUGGESTED READINGS

Blankenberg F, Wirth R, Jeffrey RB Jr, et al. Computed tomography as an adjunct to ultrasound in the diagnosis of acute acalculous cholecystitis. *Gastrointest Radiol* 1991;16:149–153.

Jeffrey RB Jr, Sommer FG. Follow-up sonography in suspected acalculous cholecystitis: preliminary clinical experience. *J Ultrasound Med* 1993;4:183–187.

Lee MS, Saini S, Brink JA, et al. Treatment of critically ill patients with sepsis of unknown cause: value of percutaneous cholecystostomy. *AJR Am J Radiol* 1991;156:1163–1166.

McDonnell CH III, Jeffrey RB Jr, Vierra M. Inflamed pericholecystic fat: color Doppler flow imaging and clinical features. *Radiology* 1994;193:547–550.

Olcott EW, Jeffrey RB Jr, Jain KA. Power versus color Doppler sonography of the normal cystic artery: implications for patients with acute cholecystitis. *AJR Am J Roentgenol* 1997;168:703–705.

Ralls PW, Colletti PM, Lapin SA, et al. Real-time sonography in suspected acute cholecystitis. *Radiology* 1985;155:767–771.

Simeone JF, Brink JA, Mueller PR, et al. The sonographic diagnosis of acute gangrenous cholecystitis: importance of the Murphy sign. *AJR Am J Radiol* 1989;152:289–290.

Teefey SA, Baron RL, Radke HM, Bigler SA. Gangrenous cholecystitis: new observations on sonography. *J Ultrasound Med* 1991;10:603–606.

12

Right Lower Quadrant Pain

Rule Out Appendicitis

R. Brooke Jeffrey, Jr.

I. CLINICAL OVERVIEW

Appendicitis is the most common cause of acute abdominal pain requiring surgery. Each year in the United States more than 250,000 surgical procedures are performed for suspected appendicitis. Before the development of cross-sectional imaging, patients with right lower quadrant pain and possible appendicitis were diagnosed and treated entirely on the basis of clinical findings. Because the symptoms of acute appendicitis can mimic a large number of other diseases, the clinical diagnosis is often imprecise. This has resulted in an accepted negative appendectomy rate of about 20%. This rate has been even higher in young adult women, often about 40%. Cross-sectional imaging with sonography and computed tomography (CT) has greatly facilitated the clinical assessment of patients with atypical signs and symptoms of appendicitis. CT and sonography can aid in establishing the diagnosis or in suggesting alternative disorders that clinically mimic appendicitis.

II. IMAGING STRATEGY

Sonography and CT are the primary imaging modalities to evaluate patients with possible acute appendicitis. The decision to perform either CT or sonography is often a matter of institutional preference and local expertise. Important factors to consider in the choice of imaging modality are the patient's body habitus and

whether perforation is considered likely. CT is preferred in obese patients and in those with suspected perforation. Sonography is the imaging method of choice during pregnancy, in pediatric patients, and in women aged 15 to 45 with normal body habitus.

III. TECHNIQUE

A. Sonography

It is important to take a brief history from the patient and to then ask the patient to point with a single finger directly to the site of maximal tenderness. This may be an important clue to an aberrantly located appendix. Graded compression sonography is performed in the right lower quadrant using a 5- to 7.5-MHz linear array transducer. The normal bowel will readily compress when light pressure is applied to the ultrasound transducer. However, the inflamed appendix will not compress. Scanning transversely in the right flank the ascending colon is first identified and followed caudally to the cecal tip. Compression is then gradually increased over the cecum to visualize the sonographic landmarks of the external iliac vessels and the psoas muscle. If these structures are not identified, the examination must be considered nondiagnostic and the patient should undergo CT.

The appendix has four constant anatomic features:

1. It originates from the cecal tip.
2. It has no peristalsis.
3. It ends in a blind pouch.
4. It has the sonographic features of bowel, namely, an inner echogenic ring representing the submucosa.

If images of the right lower quadrant are unrevealing, scans of the pelvis and upper abdomen are performed to search for an alternative diagnosis. The use of endovaginal probes provides superior imaging of adnexal structures.

B. CT

A variety of CT techniques may be used to evaluate patients for suspected appendicitis. Noncontrast CT (without oral or intravenous contrast) can be used effectively in patients who are of normal body habitus with clinically suspected uncomplicated acute appendicitis. Oral, rectal, and intravenous contrast are often essential in pediatric patients and in thin adults with little intraperitoneal fat (Fig. 1). If there is clinical suspicion of perforation or possible abscess formation, both oral and intravenous contrast should be used routinely. Intravenous contrast is injected as a uniphasic bolus at 2.5 to 3 mL/s for a total of 150 mL of 60% iodinated contrast. Scans are performed from the top of the kidneys to the symphysis pubis. With helical CT, 40-second spiral acquisitions are performed with a

pitch of 1.6 to 1. Scanning parameters include a 5-mm slice collimation. The data set is then reconstructed every 5 mm.

IV. FINDINGS

A. Sonography

The normal appendix is infrequently visualized with sonography. When it is identified, its maximal anteroposterior (AP) diameter is 5 mm or less (Fig. 2). When the maximal AP diameter of the appendix (measured from outer wall to outer wall) is 7 mm or greater and the appendix is noncompressible, the diagnosis of acute appendicitis can be established with confidence (Figs. 2–5). A 5- to 6-mm appendix represents a gray zone and clinical correlation should be advised. Appendicoliths, like calcifications in other organs, appear sonographically as echogenic foci casting acoustic shadows (see Fig. 5). Some investigators have reported that increased color Doppler flow of the appendix on color Doppler sonography indicates hyperemia and a positive study. Periappendiceal abscesses are typically hypoechoic complex fluid collections with adjacent mass effect (Fig. 6). There may be relatively little enhanced through-sound transmission due to sound absorption from proteinaceous debris within the abscess.

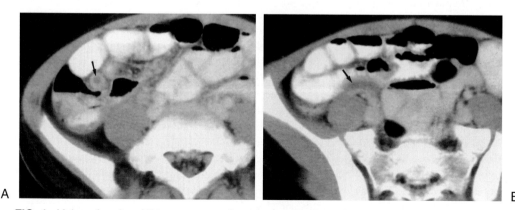

FIG. 1. Value of oral and intravenous contrast in a pediatric patient with little intraperitoneal fat. **A:** Note enhancing wall of the inflamed appendix (*arrow*). **B:** The fluid-filled lumen of the appendix is seen (*arrow*).

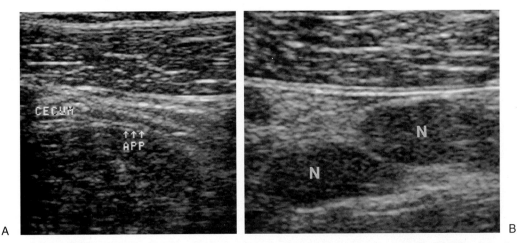

A   B

FIG. 2. Mesenteric adenitis with a normal appendix. **A:** Note the normal appendix (*APP*) originating from the cecum tip. **B:** Note the presence of multiple enlarged hypoechoic lymph nodes (*N*).

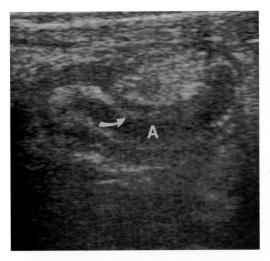
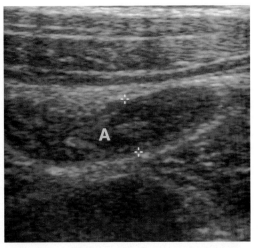

FIG. 3. Acute uncomplicated appendicitis. Note the distended, noncompressible appendix (*A*) with a preserved echogenic submucosal layer (*arrow*). The appendix measures greater than 7 mm and, therefore, is positive for acute appendicitis.

FIG. 4. Acute appendicitis with more advanced intramural inflammation. Note distended appendix (*A*) with loss of visualization of the echogenic submucosal layer.

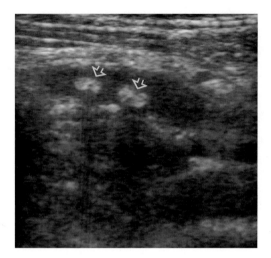

FIG. 5. Acute appendicitis with multiple appendicoliths. Note multiple echogenic foci with acoustic shadowing consistent with appendicoliths in a patient with acute appendicitis.

B. CT

Computed tomography findings in acute appendicitis include a distended appendix measuring 7 mm or more in greater AP diameter and surrounding periappendiceal inflammation (edema of the mesoappendix) (Fig. 7). A calcified appendicolith may be noted but is not a primary criterion.

V. SENSITIVITY AND SPECIFICITY

The reported sensitivity for sonography ranges from 76% to 89% with specificities of

85% to 92%. The sensitivity for CT ranges from 90% to 95% with a specificity of 92% to 96%.

VI. DIFFERENTIAL DIAGNOSIS

A. Mesenteric Adenitis

This is often a diagnosis of exclusion because enlarged mesenteric lymph nodes are a nonspecific finding. In the presence of a normal appendix, enlarged mesenteric lymph nodes demonstrated by sonography or CT suggest the diagnosis (see Fig. 1).

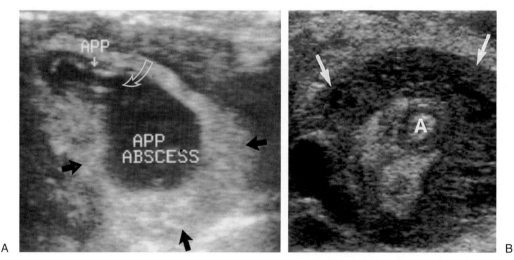

A   B

FIG. 6. Periappendiceal abscesses in two patients. In **(A)** note the hypoechoic abscess surrounded by echogenic mesenteric fat (*arrows*). The proximal normal appendix (*APP*) is identified. The site of perforation is clearly evident (*curved arrow*). In another patient **(B)** note the hypoechoic abscess (*arrows*) surrounding the appendix (*A*).

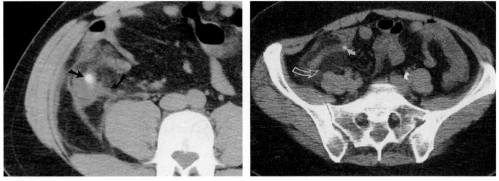

FIG. 7. Noncontrast computed tomography of an acute appendicitis in two patients. **A:** Note the calcified appendicolith (*arrow*). There is extensive surrounding inflammation from perforation (*curved arrow*). **B:** Note the appendicolith (*curved arrow*) and edema of the periappendiceal fat (*curved arrow*).

B. Infectious Ileitis and Crohn's Disease

Infectious ileitis and Crohn's disease may produce similar CT and sonographic findings with thickening of the terminal ileum with adjacent mesenteric adenopathy (Fig. 8). Crohn's disease has a greater likelihood of sinus tracts into the mesentery and abscess formation. The thickening segment of bowel typically demonstrates hyperemia with color Doppler flow.

C. Pelvic Inflammatory Disese

The most significant imaging hallmarks include evidence of either a tubo-ovarian abscess (complex cystic mass) (Figs. 9 and 10) or a dilated fallopian tube with a fluid–fluid level (pyosalpinx) (Fig. 11).

D. Cecal Diverticulitis

Paracolonic inflammatory changes are noted with mural thickening of the ascending colon and visualized diverticula.

VII. PITFALLS

A dilated right fallopian tube, a dilated right ureter (Fig. 12), and a thrombosed right gonadal

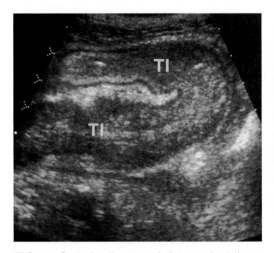

FIG. 8. Crohn's disease of the terminal ileum mimicking acute appendicitis. Note the thickened terminal ileum (*TI*) with a rigid appearance. Endoscopy revealed Crohn's disease.

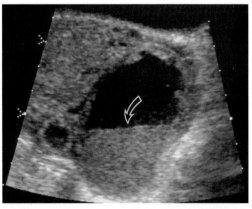

FIG. 9. Tubo-ovarian abscess. A transverse sonogram demonstrates a fluid–debris level in the left adnexa (*arrow*). The appearance is not specific and could be due to a gastrointestinal source of an abscess such as diverticulitis.

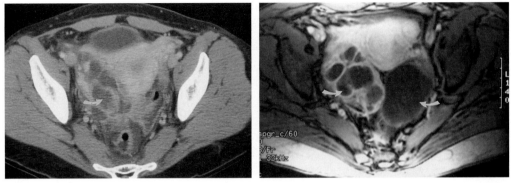

A   B

FIG. 10. Tubo-ovarian abscess on computed tomography (CT) and magnetic resonance imaging (MRI) in two patients. Contrast-enhanced CT in **(A)** demonstrates a multiseptated cystic mass in the right adnexa (*arrow*). Bilateral abscesses are noted (*arrows*) in another patient in **(B)**, seen in a gadolinium-enhanced MRI.

vein are tubular structures in the right lower quadrant that are noncompressible and could be misconstrued as an abnormal appendix. Use of endovaginal probes and scanning using full-bladder technique to evaluate the pelvic ureter can be helpful. CT is particularly valuable to evaluate a thrombosed gonadal vein. It is essential to visualize the entire length of the appendix because early appendicitis may be confined to the distal tip with a normal base of the appendix.

In Crohn's disease and tubo-ovarian abscesses, secondary inflammation of the tip of the cecum

and secondary inflammation of the appendix may occur (Fig. 13). Gas-forming infection within the appendix may cause extensive acoustic shadowing, making visualization of the appendix difficult (Fig. 14). Its lack of compressibility is an important clue to the diagnosis.

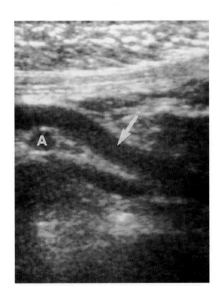

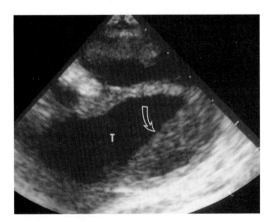

FIG. 11. Pyosalpinx. Note dilated fallopian tube (*T*) with fluid–debris level (*arrow*).

FIG. 12. Dilated ureter in the right lower quadrant mimicking appendicitis. Note the fluid-filled, noncompressible structure in the right lower quadrant (*arrow*), representing a dilated ureter. The ureters answer to the external iliac artery (*A*). A distal ureteral stone was noted.

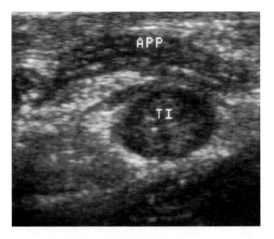

FIG. 13. Secondary inflammation of the appendix caused by Crohn's disease. Note the dilated appendix (*APP*) adjacent to the thickened and inflamed terminal ileum (*TI*). Secondary inflammation from terminal ileitis resulted in inflammatory changes within the appendix, which could have been misconstrued as primary appendicitis.

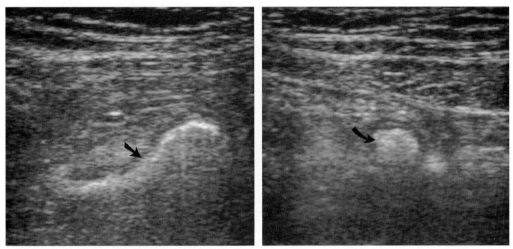

A   B

FIG. 14. Gas-filled appendix. **A:** A sagittal image of the appendix (*arrow*) is almost completely shadowed by intraluminal gas from a gas-forming infection. **B:** A small portion of the appendix (*arrow*) is identified in the region of the tip. Note the echogenic intraluminal gas.

VIII. SUGGESTED READINGS

Birnbaum BA, Jeffrey RB Jr. CT and sonographic evaluation of acute right lower quadrant abdominal pain. *AJR Am J Radiol* 1998;170:361–371.

Jeffrey RB Jr, Laing FC, Townsend RR. Acute appendicitis: sonographic criteria based on 50 cases. *Radiology* 1988; 167:327–329.

Lane MJ, Katz DS, Ross BA, Calutice-Engle TL, Mindelzun RE, Jeffrey RB Jr. Unenhanced helical CT for suspected acute appendicitis. *AJR Am J Radiol* 1997;168:405–409.

Puylaert JB. Acute appendicitis: US evaluation using graded compression. *Radiology* 1986;158:355–360.

Rioux M. Sonographic detection of the normal and abnormal appendix. *AJR Am J Radiol* 1992;158:773–788.

13

Left Lower Quadrant Pain

Rule Out Diverticulitis

Philip W. Ralls

I. CLINICAL OVERVIEW

Acute diverticulitis of the sigmoid colon is by far the most common cause of left lower quadrant pain in the adult population. Diverticulosis is present in one-third of the United States population by age 50 and approximately two-thirds by age 80. The Western diet, low in dietary grain fiber, is responsible for diverticulosis and its complications. The estimated risk of diverticulitis in the patients with diverticulosis is 10% to 25%. Symptomatic diverticulosis is usually a chronic condition characterized by left lower quadrant pain and a tender sigmoid colon on palpation. Abrupt onset of abdominal pain and alteration of bowel pattern characterize nearly all cases of diverticulitis. Localized left lower quadrant abdominal pain and tenderness may be the only symptoms in mild cases. It is often difficult to distinguish patients with mild diverticulitis from those with irritable bowel syndrome who have coincidentally discovered diverticula. Acute onset of left lower quadrant pain with fever, chills, and peritoneal signs suggests diverticulitis. Although diverticulitis generally occurs in patients 40 or more years of age, diverticulitis in the young and very elderly is often more severe and requires more aggressive therapy.

Complications of diverticulitis that require surgery or other intervention may occur in as many as 30% of patients with diverticulitis. Major complications include abscess, fistula, gastrointestinal obstruction, and perforation.

Contrast-enhanced computed tomography (CT) has revolutionized the diagnosis and treatment of diverticulitis and its complications. Contrast enema, the traditional examination to evaluate diverticulitis, is fairly accurate, but is less useful than CT in assessing pericolonic inflammation and abscess. In addition, some practitioners believe that barium or even water-soluble contrast enemas should not be performed in patients with acute diverticulitis, especially when perforation is suspected.

II. IMAGING STRATEGY

Computed tomography is the test of choice to evaluate patients with suspected complicated acute diverticulitis. Contrast enema, the traditional examination to evaluate diverticulitis, is fairly accurate, but has the drawback that it is not as good in assessing pericolonic inflammation and abscess formation. Contrast enema is the test of choice in patients with mild diverticulitis. These patients do not require emergency imaging. CT not only detects mural thickening and pericolonic inflammation, but also can be used to guide percutaneous drainage of abscesses. When abscesses are present, CT-guided abscess drainage can often eliminate multistaged surgical procedures.

Sonography can occasionally detect signs of diverticulitis, although findings are typically nonspecific. Mural thickening, increased echogenicity fat, indicative of pericolonic inflammation, and pericolonic diverticular abscesses can be seen sonographically. On occasion, extraluminal gas bubbles can be seen in association with acute diverticulitis.

III. TECHNIQUE

A. CT

Because diverticulitis is rarely an acute emergency, there is generally time for patient preparation. Oral contrast given 2 hours before scanning provides adequate colonic opacification. Oral contrast is given 30 minutes before and at the time of the study. Intravenous contrast enhancement is useful; scans prior to intravenous contrast are generally unnecessary. Helical or dynamic incremented CT are both effective. Contiguous slices of 7 to 10 mm are adequate for evaluation.

B. Contrast Enema

Some practitioners believe that contrast enema is inappropriate in patients with acute diverticulitis, mainly because of the risk of leakage and perforation. If contrast enema is performed, water-soluble contrast should be used and instilled gently with low pressure. Careful fluoroscopic monitoring is necessary. If a leak is demonstrated, the study should be terminated. Smooth muscle relaxants, such as glucagon, facilitate the examination and may reduce patient discomfort.

C. Sonography

Graded compression sonography with near-field optimized high-resolution linear array or curved array transducers can reveal wall thickening, pericolonic inflammation, and abscess. Power Doppler may reveal mural and pericolonic hyperemia.

IV. RADIOGRAPHIC FINDINGS

A. CT

Computed tomography scans in patients with acute diverticulitis may be normal or show only subtle hyperemia. Detecting diverticula is not sufficient to diagnose diverticulitis. Pericolonic inflammation is the most common CT finding (Fig. 1). It often appears as linear stranding or hazy increased density in the pericolonic fat adjacent to the site of diverticular perforation. Mural thickening, mesenteric edema, mesenteric fat inflammation, and engorged mesenteric vessels are findings of acute diverticulitis. CT findings in diverticulitis are not specific and confusion with perforated carcinoma may be a problem. Padidar and colleagues suggested that edema at the root of the sigmoid mesentery and mesenteric vascular engorgement were statistically more common in diverticulitis than in perforated carcinoma.

Extracolonic complications may occur, including abscesses (Figs. 2 and 3), free air (Figs.

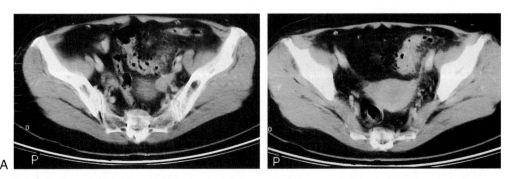

FIG. 1. Uncomplicated diverticulitis. This 58-year-old woman presented with fever and left lower quadrant pain. Computed tomography findings (**A** and **B**) are indicative of uncomplicated acute diverticulitis. Note the diverticula, mild wall thickening, and pericolonic inflammation. No abscess formation is seen.

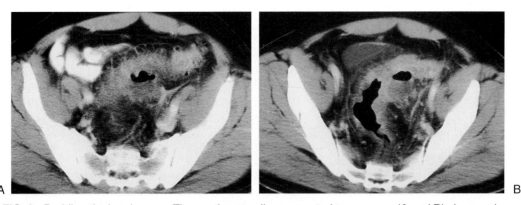

FIG. 2. Peridiverticular abscess. The contiguous slice computed tomograms (**A** and **B**) show pericolonic inflammation and an abscess dorsal to the distal sigmoid colon. An air–fluid level is seen in the abscess on the more caudal image.

4 and 5) from perforation into the peritoneal space, fistulae, or ureteral obstruction. Pyelophlebitis (septic portal venous thrombosis) and associated liver abscess may occur (Fig. 6 and Color Plate 4).

B. Contrast Enema

On contrast enema, diverticulitis usually is detected as deformed diverticular sacs, a mass

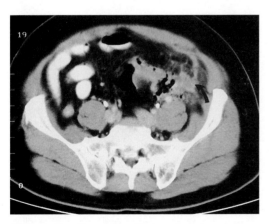

FIG. 3. Small peridiverticular abscess. A computed tomography scan in the pelvis shows diverticulitis with perforation, pericolonic inflammation, and a small pericolonic abscess (*curved arrow*). Perforation with abscess formation is one of the most common complications of acute diverticulitis. A lesion this small probably does not require percutaneous drainage, unless it is unresponsive to conservative management.

effect because of an abscess or inflammatory mass, and extravasation of water-soluble contrast material. Spasm and near obstruction may also occur. Sinus tracts running to the urinary bladder, other bowel loops, the skin, or elsewhere may occur in diverticulitis.

C. Sonography

Sonography is often the first examination requested in patients with abdominal pain. Yacoe and colleagues described the following sonographic findings in diverticulitis: mural thickening, increased echogenicity of inflamed mesenteric fat, and extraluminal air bubbles. Power Doppler may reveal mural and pericolonic hyperemia (Fig. 7 and Color Plate 5).

V. SENSITIVITY AND SPECIFICITY

Sensitivity of CT for diverticulitis is 80% to 100%. In a study by Cho and colleagues of 56 patients with diverticulitis, CT suggested an alternative diagnosis in 20 of 29 patients who did not have diverticulitis, whereas barium enema identified only 3 of those patients.

Contrast enema, the traditional examination to evaluate diverticulitis, has a sensitivity of 60% to 90% for sigmoid diverticulitis.

No good data are available for the sensitivity and specificity of sonography in the diagnosis of acute diverticulitis. Although our experience suggests that CT is superior to sonography in

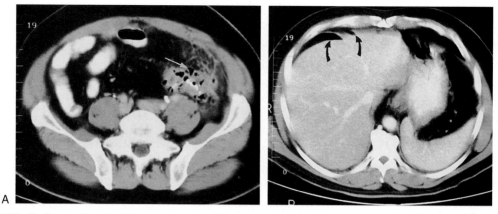

FIG. 4. Acute diverticulitis with free air from a perforation. **A:** A computed tomography (CT) scan done through the upper pelvic region reveals severe diverticulitis with mural thickening, pericolonic inflammation, and a narrow lumen (see contrast within it). Note the likely region of perforation (*arrow*). **B:** A CT scan near the diaphragm shows air in the infradiaphragmatic region (*curved arrows*). Perforation into the peritoneal cavity is an unusual complication of diverticulitis. Usually the perforation is walled off by the inflammatory process, and localized abscess results.

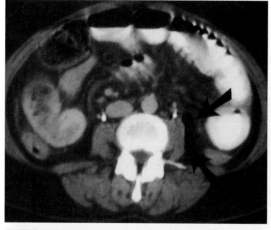

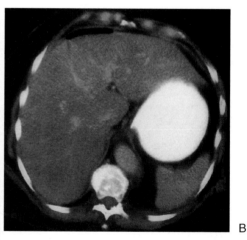

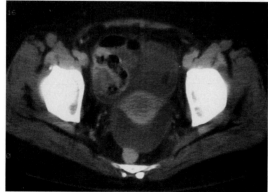

FIG. 5. Perforated sigmoid diverticulitis. Computed tomography of the midabdomen **(A)** shows air adjacent to the psoas muscle. This gas arose from a perforated diverticulum. A scan in the same patient higher in the abdomen **(B)** shows free air in the intraperitoneal cavity, ventral to the liver. This patient also had a large pelvic abscess **(C)**, the most common complication of diverticulitis.

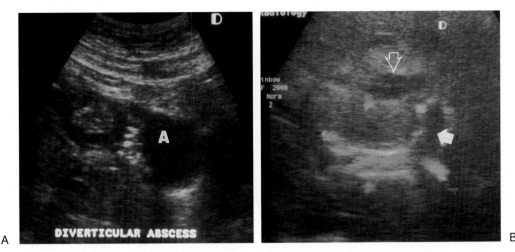

FIG. 6. Diverticulitis with pylephlebitis liver abscess. An oblique sonogram through the left lower quadrant **(A)** reveals a minimally thickened bowel loop with a contiguous diverticular abscess (*A*). A transverse color Doppler sonogram **(B)** through the porta hepatis of the liver shows thrombosis of the left portal vein (*arrow*) and a liver abscess (*open arrow*). This is an example of septic portal venous thrombosis (pylephlebitis) caused by diverticulitis. Pylephlebitis is associated with a very high prevalence of liver abscess, as exemplified by this case. (See also Color Plate 4.)

acute diverticulitis, Pradel et al., in a study performed in Montpellier, France, suggested that sonography and CT can have similar accuracy in patients with suspected acute diverticulitis.

VI. DIFFERENTIAL DIAGNOSIS

A. Perforated Colon Carcinoma

The symptoms of diverticular disease and perforated colonic carcinoma may be similar. The ra-

diologic differentiation is often difficult or impossible; perforated colon carcinoma may be totally indistinguishable from acute diverticulitis on imaging. A shouldered or "apple core"-like mass, rather than more diffuse irregular thickening, suggests the diagnosis of carcinoma (Fig. 8). Muscle hypertrophy, fibrosis, edema, intramural inflammation, or an organizing intramural inflammatory mass suggests diverticulitis rather than colon carcinoma. In addition, edema fluid in

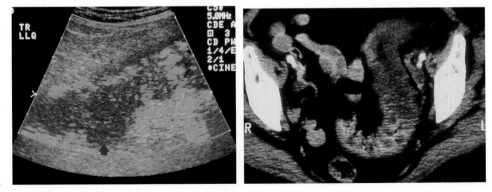

FIG. 7. Focal ischemia and diffuse inflammation from diverticulitis. This oblique power Doppler sonogram **(A)** shows mural and pericolonic hyperemia manifest as color-coded flow. This corresponds to inflammation. Note the ischemic area of decreased flow (*arrow*). (See also Color Plate 5.) The corresponding CT scan **(B)** likewise shows mural thickening.

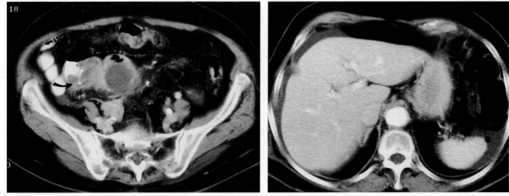

FIG. 8. Diverticulitis and peridiverticular abscess simulate perforated colon carcinoma. A computed tomography (CT) scan through the pelvis **(A)** reveals an abscess and a contiguous apparent mass in the sigmoid colon (*arrow*). Relatively little pericolonic inflammation was present in this patient. A CT scan through the upper abdomen **(B)** shows free fluid. The initial diagnosis was perforated sigmoid colon carcinoma with abscess. This proved to be diverticulitis with rupture, not colon carcinoma.

the root of the mesentery vascular engorgement is statistically more common in diverticulitis.

B. Infectious Colitis

Infectious colitis can, on occasion, clinically mimic diverticulitis. Findings on CT are generally quite different, however, consisting of diffuse bowel

wall thickening, usually with relatively little extra-colonic abnormality (Figs. 9 and 10; Color Plate 6).

C. Crohn's Disease

Crohn's disease typically involves the distal small bowel. It may, however, involve any area of the gastrointestinal tract including the colon

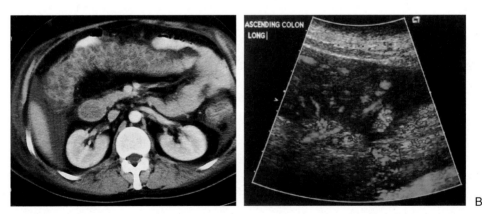

FIG. 9. Psuedomembranous colitis. The computed tomography scan **(A)** shows a thickened colonic wall with low attenuation and some areas of linear enhancement throughout the wall. Ascites is present. Power Doppler **(B)** in the same location shows hyperemia of the wall. (See also Color Plate 6.)

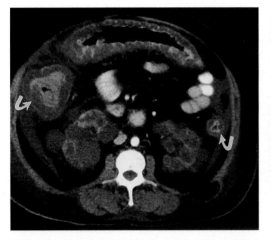

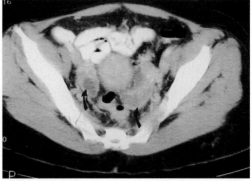

FIG. 12. Pelvic inflammatory disease simulates diverticulitis clinically. This patient presented with left lower quadrant pain and was suspected of having diverticulitis. Computed tomography shows no evidence of pericolonic abnormalities, but shows what is likely a right-sided tubo-ovarian abscess and a left-sided pyosalpinx (*arrows*).

FIG. 10. *Clostridium difficile* colitis. This patient with polycystic disease presented with acute left lower quadrant pain. This is atypical for *C. difficile* colitis (pseudomembranous enterocolitis). Note the edematous wall of the ascending transverse and descending colon (*arrows*). A moderate amount of ascitic fluid is present. Colitis related to *C. difficile* more typically presents with right lower pain than with left lower quadrant pain.

(Fig. 11). Crohn's disease is characterized by wall thickening from edema, fibrosis inflammation, and lymphatic obstruction. CT can identify inflamed segments of bowel. The most frequent CT finding is hyperemia—homogeneously enhancing the bowel wall. Complications include strictures, mesenteric abnormalities, inflammation, adenopathy, fistulae (in up to one-third of

patients), sinus tracts, neoplasm, renal and kidney stones, and sacroiliitis. Hyperemia may be noted on CT and power Doppler. Theoretically, isolated left colonic Crohn's disease might simulate acute diverticulitis. As a practical matter, however, Crohn's disease is differentiated from diverticulitis because of its predilection to involve the small bowel and a typical history.

D. Other

Other fairly common causes of left lower quadrant pain and fever include pelvic inflammatory disease (Figs. 12 and 13), gastrointesti-

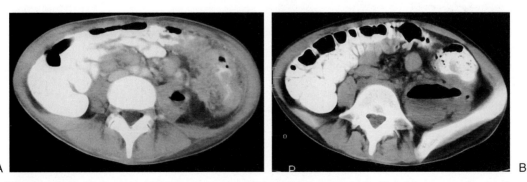

A   B

FIG. 11. Crohn's disease with psoas abscess. This patient presented with left lower quadrant pain and was clinically thought to have diverticulitis. The markedly irregular left colon with wall thickening **(A)** is clearly abnormal, but the findings are nonspecific. Note the psoas abscess with air–fluid level within it (*arrow*). **B:** Subsequent biopsy proved this to be colonic Crohn's disease.

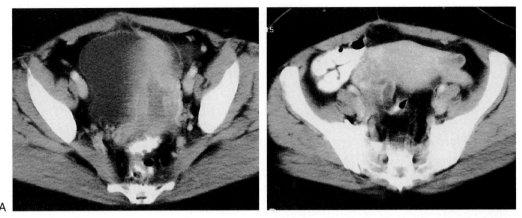

A   B

FIG. 13. Left lower quadrant pain in pelvic inflammatory disease. The computed tomography scan **(A)** in a 39-year-old woman reveals a dilated endometrial cavity with left adnexal/left lower quadrant inflammation. Dilated tubes are seen bilaterally **(B)**. Pelvic inflammatory disease is one condition that can mimic acute diverticulitis.

nal ischemia (Fig. 14), volvulus, and nephrolithiasis.

VII. PITFALLS

There are very few causes of left lower quadrant pain that simulate diverticulitis. Perforated colon carcinoma, however, may be essentially impossible to distinguish from diverticulitis (see Fig. 8).

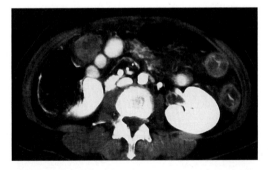

FIG. 14. Ischemic colitis. This 75-year-old woman presented with fever and left lower quadrant pain. The findings show edema of the bowel wall with low attenuation strongly suggestive of ischemic colitis. There is some increased density in the pericolonic fat.

VIII. SUGGESTED READINGS

Balthazar EJ, Megibow AJ, Schinella RA, Gordon R. Limitations in the CT diagnosis of acute diverticulitis: comparison of CT, contrast enema, and pathologic findings in 16 patients. *AJR Am J Roentgenol* 1990;154:281–285.

Cho KC, Morehouse HT, Alterman DD, Thornhill BA. Sigmoid diverticulitis: diagnostic role of CT—comparison with barium enema studies. *Radiology* 1990;176:111–115.

Hulnick DH, Megibow AJ, Balthazar EJ, Naidich DP, Bosniak MA. Computed tomography in the evaluation of diverticulitis. *Radiology* 1984;152:491–495.

Padidar AM, Jeffrey RB Jr, Mindelzun RE, Dolph JF. Differentiating sigmoid diverticulitis from carcinoma on CT scans: mesenteric inflammation suggests diverticulitis. *AJR Am J Roentgenol* 1994;163:81–83.

Pradel JA, Adell JF, Taourel P, Djafari M, Monnin-Delhom E, Bruel JM. Acute colonic diverticulitis: prospective comparative evaluation with US and CT. *Radiology* 1997;205:503–512.

Yacoe ME, Jeffrey RB Jr. Sonography of appendicitis and diverticulitis. *Radiol Clin North Am* 1994;32:899–912.

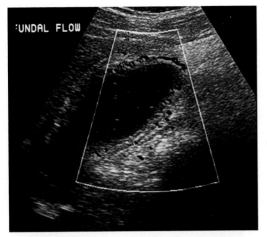

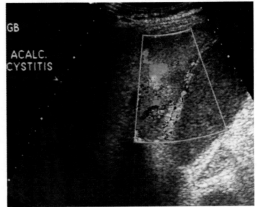

COLOR PLATE 1. Gangrenous acalculous cholecystitis with fundal flow on power Doppler. This patient presented with right upper quadrant pain, fever, and a normal white cell count. Prominent fundal flow was present on both power and color Doppler. Although more common in acute cholecystitis, normal fundal flow is now often seen because of the improved sensitivity of newer Doppler systems. (See also Chapter 11, Figure 4B.)

COLOR PLATE 2. 5 Acute acalculous cholecystitis with increased mural flow. The color Doppler sonogram shows flow in the cystic artery throughout the wall. These findings, in the correct clinical setting, suggest acute acalculous cholecystitis. (See also Chapter 11, Figure 5B.)

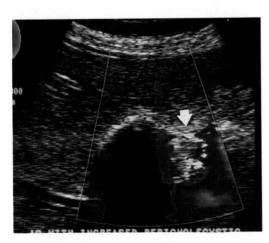

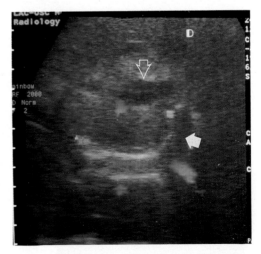

COLOR PLATE 3. Acute cholecystitis with increased flow in inflamed fat. The transverse power Doppler sonogram shows increased flow in the echogenic, inflamed fat (*arrow*) medial to the gallbladder. Echogenic fat with increased flow supports the diagnosis of acute cholecystitis. (See also Chapter 11, Figure 13B.)

COLOR PLATE 4. Diverticulitis with pyelophlebitis with liver abscess. A transverse color Doppler sonogram through the porta hepatis of the liver shows thrombosis of the left portal vein (*arrow*) and a liver abscess (*open arrow*). This is an example of septic portal venous thrombosis (pyelophlebitis) caused by diverticulitis. Pyelophlebitis is associated with a very high prevalence of liver abscess, as exemplified by this case. (See also Chapter 13, Figure 6B.)

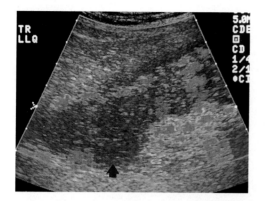

COLOR PLATE 5. Focal ischemia and diffuse inflammation from diverticulitis. This oblique power Doppler sonogram **(A)** shows mural and pericolonic hyperemia manifest as color-coded flow. This corresponds to inflammation. Note the ischemic area of decreased flow (*arrow*). (See also Chapter 13, Figure 7A.)

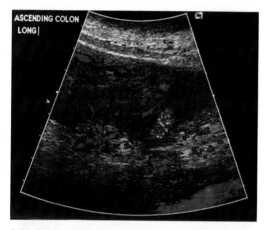

COLOR PLATE 6. Psuedomembranous colitis. Power Doppler shows hyperemia of the wall. (See also Chapter 13, Figure 9B.)

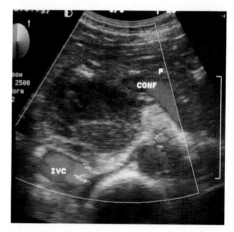

COLOR PLATE 7. Tuberculous abscess. This patient presented with fever and abdominal pain. The masslike primarily hypoechoic abscess was detected in the juxtapancreatic region. After aspiration, this proved to be a tuberculous abscess. IVC, inferior vena cava; CONF, confluence of splenic and superior mesenteric veins; p, pancreas. (See also Chapter 16, Figure 8.)

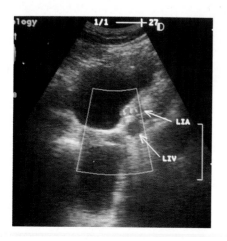

COLOR PLATE 8. Pelvic lymphoceles. This patient presented 3 weeks after pelvic surgery with a low-grade fever and pelvic pain. This fluid collection is just medial to the iliac vessels. This is the typical appearance and location for a lymphocele, although the lesion was aspirated to exclude the possibility of abscess. Another lymphocele is seen deep to the lesion contiguous with the iliac vessel. LIV, left iliac vein; LIA, left iliac artery. (See also Chapter 16, Figure 9.)

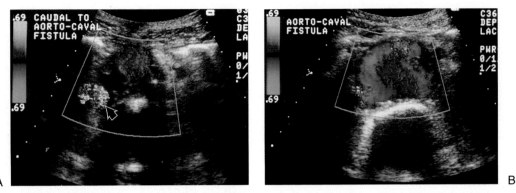

A   B

COLOR PLATE 9. Aortic aneurysm with a portocaval fistula. Transverse sonogram **(A)** shows a small aortic aneurysm with a perianeurysmal hematoma. Note that the inferior vena cava (*open arrow*) is only slightly dilated in this image obtained caudal to the site of the fistula. A sonogram near the site of the aortocaval fistula **(B)** shows marked dilatation of the inferior vena cava with turbulent flow. This patient presented with mild congestive heart failure related to the arteriovenous shunting. The exact site of the aortocaval fistula could not be demonstrated sonographically. (See also Chapter 17, Figure 1.)

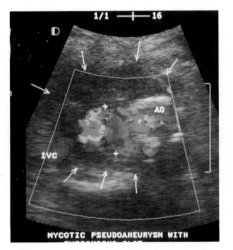

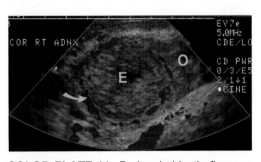

COLOR PLATE 10. Ruptured mycotic abdominal aortic aneurysm. This 56-year-old user of intravenous drugs presented with a sudden onset of lower abdominal back pain and hypotension. Color flow sonography revealed a calcified aorta with a mycotic abdominal aortic aneurysm between the inferior vena cava (*IVC*) and aorta (*AO*). (See also Chapter 17, Figure 3A.)

COLOR PLATE 11. Peritrophoblastic flow surrounding ectopic pregnancy. Note the echogenic ring of an ectopic pregnancy (*E*) adjacent to the right ovary. Power Doppler demonstrates peritrophoblastic flow around the ectopic gestation (*curved arrow*). (See also Chapter 19, Figure 11.)

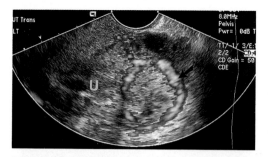

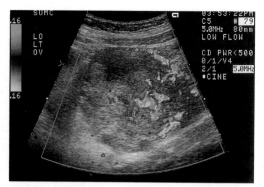

COLOR PLATE 12. Coronal (interstitial) ectopic pregnancy with peritrophoblastic flow. Endovaginal scan of the uterus demonstrates peritrophoblastic flow around the coronal ectopic gestation along the left lateral marginal of the uterus (*U*). (See also Chapter 19, Figure 13.)

COLOR PLATE 14. Reperfusion of a torsed ovary following detorsion. This patient had severe left lower quadrant pain that suddenly subsided. A color Doppler image of the left ovary demonstrates an enlarged ovary with prominent internal flow. Over a period of several weeks, the ovary reduced in size. This likely represents detorsion with associated increased profusion. (See also Chapter 20, Figure 5.)

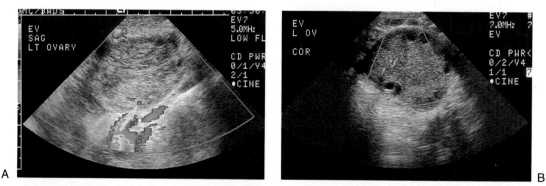

A   B

COLOR PLATE 13. Torsed ovary with preserved arterial flow in two patients. **A:** Note the enlarged echogenic left ovary with peripheral color Doppler signals still evident (*arrow*). Low-amplitude arterial waveforms were obtained from this small vessel. **B:** In another patient, the preserved arterial flow is more centrally within the torsed left ovary on this endovaginal color Doppler. No central venous flow was obtained. (See also Chapter 20, Figure 4.)

14

Acute Abdominal Pain

Rule Out Acute Pancreatitis

R. Brooke Jeffrey, Jr.

I. CLINICAL OVERVIEW

Computed tomography (CT) is often a valuable tool for the evaluation and management of patients with acute pancreatitis. When the diagnosis is in doubt, characteristic CT findings may confirm acute pancreatitis or suggest an alternative diagnosis, such as bowel obstruction, perforated ulcer, or mesenteric ischemia. Contrast-enhanced CT is essential for the early diagnosis of complications of pancreatitis such as necrosis, abscess formation, or hemorrhage. Early diagnosis of complications with prompt surgical or percutaneous intervention has been a key factor in improving survival in patients with severe pancreatitis.

II. IMAGING STRATEGY

Patients with necrotizing pancreatitis often present clinically with an elevated Ranson or APACHE (Acute Physiology and Chronic Health Evaluation) score. There is a greater likelihood of complications in these patients, and therefore, CT should be performed early in the clinical course. Contrast-enhanced magnetic resonance imaging may be used as an alternative to CT in patients with renal insufficiency or allergy to iodinated contrast. Sonography plays a secondary role in the initial assessment of patients with possible pancreatitis. Gallbladder sonography may prove valuable in confirming gallstones or common duct stones in gallstone pancreatitis.

III. TECHNIQUE

Computed tomography is performed both with and without intravenous contrast. Unenhanced scans are helpful to diagnose hemorrhage by identifying peripancreatic high-attenuation fluid [more than 35 Hounsfield units (HU)] (Fig. 1). Contrast-enhanced scans are essential to assess the extent of pancreatic necrosis, which is diagnosed as an area of nonenhancing (avascular) parenchyma (Fig. 2). Scan collimation is 7 to 8 mm for both unenhanced and enhanced scans. If possible, breath-held helical acquisitions are performed. If significant pancreatic hemorrhage is identified on noncontrast scans, a biphasic protocol may be used to identify a peripancreatic pseudoaneurysm. If no hemorrhage is identified, a single acquisition is performed from the diaphragm to below the pancreas during the portal venous phase using a 60- to 70-second delay and a uniphasic bolus injection of 150 mL of 60% contrast injected at 3 mL/s. A pitch (1 to 1.5) is used.

For the biphasic protocol the injection rate is increased to 4 to 5 mL/s. The arterial phase images of the pancreas are obtained after a 25-second delay using a 5-mm collimation. A 30-second helical scan is performed with a breath-hold. Following the arterial phase the patient breathes freely for 10 to 15 seconds and is then repositioned for the venous phase acquisition, which is identical to the previously described uniphasic venous phase scanning protocol using a 7-mm collimation and sufficient pitch to cover the abdomen and pelvis.

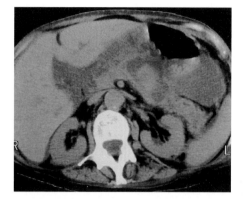

FIG. 1. Noncontrast computed tomography demonstrating pancreatic hemorrhage. Note the high attenuation clot within the area of pancreatic necrosis (*arrow*) in the body of the pancreas.

IV. FINDINGS

Patients with acute pancreatitis fall into two broad pathologic categories: edematous pancreatitis and necrotizing pancreatitis. Edematous pancreatitis is the much milder form of the disease, with substantially lower morbidity and mortality. However, it is possible for initial edematous pancreatitis to evolve into necrotizing pancreatitis later in the patient's clinical course. Necrotizing pancreatitis refers to glandular necrosis and fat saponification that occur

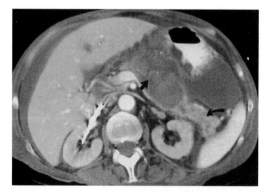

FIG. 2. Contrast-enhanced computed tomography of pancreatic necrosis. Note the large area of necrosis in the body of the pancreas anterior to the splenic vein (*arrow*). There is normal enhancement of the tail of the pancreas (*curved arrow*).

when activated proteolytic enzymes such as trypsin extravasate from the pancreatic duct and affect the pancreatic parenchyma in patients with necrotizing pancreatitis surrounding retroperitoneal tissues. These patients are prone to hemorrhage, abscess formation, and pseudocysts.

In selected patients with edematous pancreatitis, there may be little obvious CT abnormality. Subtle enlargement of the gland may be the only finding. There may be mild soft tissue infiltration or fluid in the peripancreatic spaces such as the anterior pararenal space (Fig. 3). In the absence of necrosis, the pancreatic parenchyma enhances uniformly with intravenous contrast and there are no avascular areas of low attenuation.

Characteristic features of necrotizing pancreatitis on CT include demonstration of peripancreatic hemorrhage on noncontrast CT and areas of lack of enhancement with intravenous contrast consistent with avascular necrosis (Fig. 4). Peripancreatic fluid collections are common in necrotizing pancreatitis and may be located anywhere from the mediastinum to the groin. However, the most common sites of fluid collection include the pararenal spaces, the lesser sac, and the transverse mesocolon (Fig. 5). The term "acute fluid collection" should be used in the acute phase of the disease before the development of encapsulated fluid collections or pseudocysts that are typically seen 6 to 12 weeks after an acute attack of necrotizing pancreatitis. Pseudocysts demonstrate mass effect and have a clearly visible enhancing fibrous wall (Fig. 6).

The most serious complication of necrotizing pancreatitis is the development of infected pancreatic necrosis. Because most patients with necrotizing pancreatitis have fever and leukocytosis, it is difficult to clinically distinguish patients with sterile necrosis from those with infected necrosis. One of the main values of CT is to guide needle-directed aspiration to make an early diagnosis of this entity. Prompt surgical intervention is usually required for infected necrosis with wide pancreatic débridement. Gas bubbles (emphysematous pancreatitis) may be clearly visible in CT in patients with gas-forming infection. Pseudoaneurysms may present with hemorrhage into a pancreatic

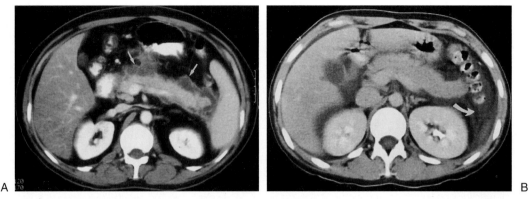

FIG. 3. Edematous pancreatitis on contrast computed tomography. **A:** Note normal-enhancing pancreatic parenchyma with small peripancreatic fluid collections (*arrows*). **B:** Note the normal-appearing enhancing pancreas with soft tissue infiltration in the left anterior space (*arrow*).

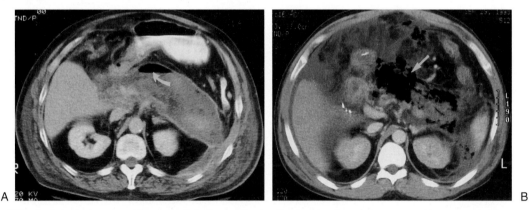

FIG. 4. Infected pancreatic necrosis in two patients. Contrast-enhanced computed tomography demonstrates virtual complete lack of enhancement of the pancreatic parenchyma. **A:** Note the air–fluid level in the region of the body of the pancreas due to infected pancreatic necrosis (*arrow*). In another patient **(B)**, note extensive gas-forming infection within the pancreas (*arrow*).

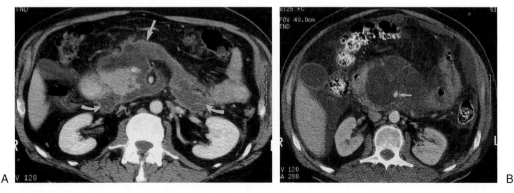

FIG. 5. Peripancreatic fluid collections caused by necrotizing pancreatitis. **A:** Note the multiple fluid collections involving the transverse mesocolon (*arrow*) and bilateral anterior pararenal spaces (*curved arrows*). **B:** Note the large pancreatic fluid collection stemming from the head of the pancreas and involving the root of the small bowel mesentery. Note the encasement of the superior mesentery artery (*arrow*) by the fluid.

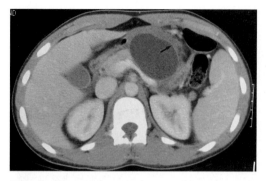

FIG. 6. Pancreatic pseudocysts. Note the well-defined fluid collection in the body of the pancreas with an enhancing fibrous capsule (*arrows*).

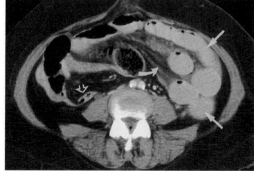

FIG. 7. Small bowel obstruction clinically mimicking acute appendicitis. Note dilated loops of proximal small bowel (*arrows*) with tethered mesentery and hemorrhage within the mesentery (*curved arrow*). The collapse of the distal small bowel (*open arrow*) is indicative of small bowel obstruction.

pseudocyst or in the adjacent retroperitoneum. Contrast enhancement is central for precise diagnosis of pseudoaneurysms. In selected patients, however, when CT is negative, angiography may be required in those with ongoing hemorrhage. Angiography may be both diagnostic and therapeutic because peripancreatic pseudoaneurysms can be embolized with a high degree of success.

V. SENSITIVITY AND SPECIFICITY

Patients with edematous pancreatitis may have few or no changes on CT. Patients with biliary pancreatitis may have marked elevation of serum amylase with abdominal pain yet have an unremarkable CT. CT is highly reliable for pancreatic and peripancreatic changes of necrotizing pancreatitis, which are typically not subtle in nature.

VI. DIFFERENTIAL DIAGNOSIS

In patients with characteristic CT features of pancreatitis including abnormal parenchymal enhancement and peripancreatic fluid collections or hemorrhage, the CT diagnosis is reliable. Other retroperitoneal inflammatory processes such as perforated ulcers, diverticulitis, or even appendicitis do not generally cause intrinsic abnormalities of the pancreas. Patients with cholecystitis, bowel obstruction, or bowel

perforation may clinically be misdiagnosed as having necrotizing pancreatitis (Figs. 7, 8, and 9). On occasion, other retroperitoneal disorders such as perforated ulcers or diverticulitis may result in peripancreatic inflammatory changes, but in general, these are not diagnostic dilemmas.

VII. PITFALLS

A small subset of patients with pancreatic carcinoma may have a rupture in the main pancreatic duct and present with a clinical syndrome

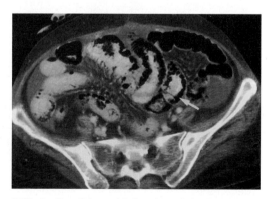

FIG. 8. Small bowel infarction clinically mimicking acute pancreatitis. Note extensive small bowel pneumatosis from infarction (*arrow*).

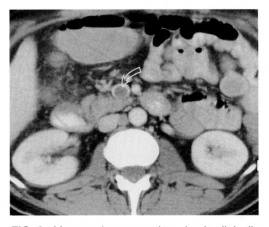

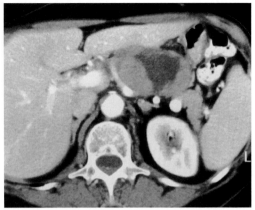

FIG. 9. Mesenteric venous thrombosis clinically mimicking acute pancreatitis. Patient presented with abdominal pain and elevated amylase level. Note thrombus in superior mesenteric vein (*arrow*).

FIG. 11. Cystic pancreatic metastases mimicking pancreatic pseudocysts. A cystic metastasis on the body of the pancreas from ovarian carcinoma is noted (*arrow*).

confused with acute pancreatitis (Fig. 10). Primary or metastatic cystic pancreatic tumors may be misdiagnosed as postinflammatory pseudocysts (Fig. 11). Peripancreatic masses such as lymphoma may at times mimic pancreatitis, but generally there are no associated fluid collections and the clinical presentation is quite different.

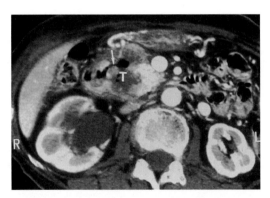

FIG. 10. Pancreatic carcinoma invading the duodenum clinically presenting as acute pancreatitis. Note the hypoattenuating tumor in the head of the pancreas (*T*). The tumor has eroded into the duodenum with a gas collection contiguous with the lumen of the duodenum (*arrow*). The patient had an elevated amylase level and abdominal pain. Surgery revealed pancreatic carcinoma invading the duodenum.

VIII. REFERENCES

Balthazar EJ, Robinson DL, Megibow AJ, et al. Acute pancreatitis: value of CT in establishing prognosis. *Radiology* 1990;174:331–336.

Jeffrey RB Jr, Grendell JH, Federle MP, et al. Improved survival with early CT diagnosis of pancreatic abscess. *Gastrointest Radiol* 1987;12:26–30.

Kemppainen E, Sainio V, Haapiainen R, et al. Early localization of necrosis by contrast-enhanced computed tomography can predict outcome in severe acute pancreatitis. *Br J Surg* 1996;83:924–929.

Ranson JH. Diagnostic standards for acute pancreatitis. *World J Surg* 1997;21(2):136–142.

Yassa NA, Agostini JT, Ralls PW. Accuracy of CT in estimating extent of pancreatic necrosis. *Clin Imaging* 1997; 12:407–410.

15

Crampy Abdominal Pain

Rule Out Small Bowel Obstruction

Philip W. Ralls

I. CLINICAL OVERVIEW

Obstruction of the small bowel is one of the most common causes of abdominal pain requiring surgery. Adhesions (Fig. 1), usually related to previous surgery, are the most common cause of small bowel obstruction (75%). Other extrinsic causes of small bowel obstruction include malignant tumor and hernia (Fig. 2). Intrinsic causes are less frequent and include neoplasm, inflammatory bowel disease, ischemic bowel disease, and intussusception (Fig. 3 and Table 1). Bowel obstruction typically causes pain, vomiting, distention, and constipation. Vomiting is more common with more proximal small bowel obstruction, whereas distention predominates in patients with more distal obstruction. When strangulation occurs, ischemia and necrosis may eventuate. The pain becomes greater and more continuous. Tenderness to palpation, guarding, leukocytosis, fever, and heart rate of greater than 100 beats/min are signs of bowel strangulation.

Small bowel obstruction can often be diagnosed clinically and with abdominal radiographs (anteroposterior and decubitus or upright films). It has been estimated that plain film findings are diagnostic in about 50% to 60% of patients, equivocal in about 20% to 30%, and normal, nonspecific, or misleading in 10% to 20%. Frager and colleagues found that the sensitivity of plain films was 46%, and that of computed tomography (CT) was 100%. They concluded that CT should be used when the results of clinical and plain film evaluation are inconclusive. CT is useful to differentiate adynamic ileus from obstruction and may be helpful in the diagnosis of strangulated (ischemic) obstruction. In the study by Taourel and co-workers, CT correctly distinguished between small bowel obstruction and ileus in 98% of the patients. CT was able to identify strangulation in 75% of patients with proven strangulation. CT enabled the authors to modify an erroneous clinical diagnosis correctly in 21% of cases, changing management in those patients.

Sonography can likewise detect dilated bowel loops, especially when they are fluid filled. Sonography can also delineate the site of obstruction and assess bowel ischemia. It is more technically demanding than CT and plays a limited role in assessing these patients.

II. IMAGING STRATEGY

In patients with a typical clinical presentation, an abdominal series with classic findings is sufficient for diagnosis. Gupta and Dupuy, in a review of imaging of the acute abdomen, stated that plain film radiography should be the first imaging study for suspected cases of bowel perforation or obstruction. When plain film findings are not diagnostic, CT scanning is appropriate. CT shows the level of obstruction by identifying a transition from dilated to nondilated bowel. In most patients, the cause of obstruction can be identified (Figs. 3 and 4). A major advantage of CT is its ability to identify the cause of obstruc-

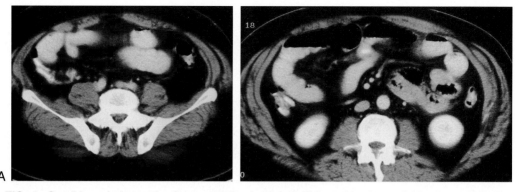

A   B

FIG. 1. Small bowel obstruction from an adhesive band. This patient has a fairly abrupt transition from dilated to nondilated bowel in the distal ileum **(A)**. Images obtained at a higher level **(B)** show dilatation of the proximal small bowel with air–fluid levels. Note the nondistended colon. Despite the fact that the patient had not had previous surgery and had no history suggestive of abdominal pathology, this obstruction was related to an adhesion in the right lower abdomen.

tion in many patients and to diagnose strangulation and other complications of small bowel obstruction.

Sonography has been used successfully in evaluating patients with small bowel obstruction, although limitations related to bowel gas make it less useful than CT. One advantage of real-time sonography is that it can detect hyperperistalsis associated with small bowel obstruction. Contrast enemas, which diagnose small bowel obstruction by identifying a collapsed ileum, are rarely used.

III. TECHNIQUE

A. Plain Films

The plain films obtained for evaluation of patients with suspected small bowel obstruction should include a supine abdominal film and

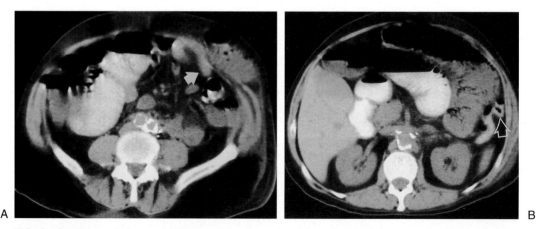

A   B

FIG. 2. Small bowel obstruction from an incisional hernia. **A:** A computed tomography scan at the level of the ventral hernia reveals dilated small bowel in the subcutaneous area. The contiguous nondilated bowel (*arrow*) demonstrates the point of transition at the level of the abdominal wall hernia. **B:** A scan at a higher level shows multiple loops of dilated small bowel with air–fluid levels and the nondilated splenic flexure (*open arrow*).

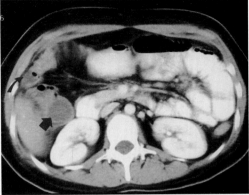

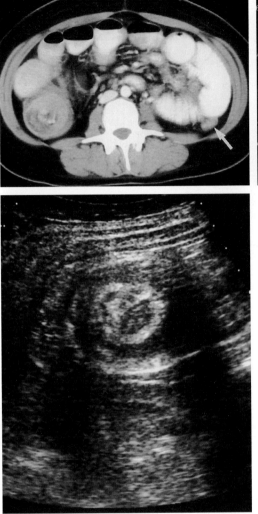

FIG. 3. Intussusception from an inflammatory polyp. This patient presented with small bowel obstruction because of intussusception. A computed tomography (CT) scan through the midabdomen **(A)** reveals dilated loops of small bowel and a collapsed left colon (*arrow*). The ileocolic intussusception is seen on the right (*open arrow*). Note the central intussuscipiens surrounded by fat within the colonic intussusceptum. A transverse sonogram near the same level **(B)** shows similar findings, with echogenic fat representing the mesenteric fat associated with the intussuscipiens. A CT scan of the high level **(C)** shows the inflammatory polyp that was the leading edge for the intussusceptum (*arrow*). Notice the dilated loops of small bowel and the nondilated hepatic flexure (*curved arrow*).

either an upright or decubitus abdominal film. Optimally, the patient should be upright or decubitus for 5 minutes before the film is obtained.

B. CT

Both oral and intravenous contrast are useful in patients with suspected small bowel obstruction. Water-soluble oral contrast with a 2% iodine concentration is best. Barium preparations are less desirable because of concerns about strangulation and leakage from the gastrointestinal tract. Iodinated contrast (150 mL) should be injected at a rate of 2 to 3 mL/s. Scanning should

TABLE 1. *Common causes of small bowel obstruction*

Extrinsic	Intrinsic
Adhesion	Crohn's Disease
Malignancy	Intussusception
External Hernia	Radiation Stricture
Internal Hernia	Foreign Body
Volvulus	Mesenteric Ischemia
Abscess	
Hematoma	

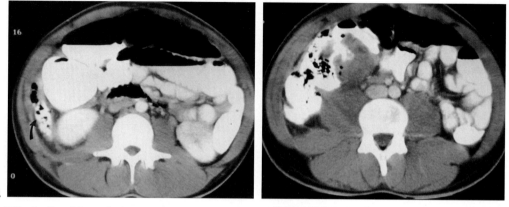

FIG. 4. Small bowel obstruction related to mesenteric hematoma. A computed tomography (CT) scan **(A)** through the midabdomen shows multiple dilated loops of small bowel with air–fluid levels. The right colon is collapsed (*arrow*). A CT scan at the lower level **(B)** reveals a mesenteric mass at the point of transition. Note the nondilated small bowel to the right of the mass and the dilated small bowel to the left. The nature of the mass was not determined at the time of CT. The patient gave no significant history for trauma. At surgery, there was tissue disruption and a hematoma causing bowel obstruction.

commence after a 60-second delay. Spiral scans should be performed to encompass the entire abdomen using an 8- to 10-mm collimation and a pitch of 1.5 with reconstruction at 10-mm intervals. If spiral scanning is not available, 10-mm collimated and incremented dynamic scans are appropriate throughout the abdomen and pelvis.

C. Sonography

Sonography using graded compression with high-resolution linear array transducers may identify abnormal hyperperistalsis, the transition from dilated to nondilated bowel, and also the cause of obstruction.

IV. RADIOGRAPHIC FINDINGS

A. Plain Films

Plain film findings diagnostic for small bowel obstruction (Fig. 5) include gaseous or fluid distention (2.5 cm or greater diameter) of small bowel loops relative to the colon or other segments of the small bowel. Air–fluid levels in the dilated small bowel segments are characteristic on the upright or decubitus abdominal film. Fluid-filled loops are clearly harder to appreciate

and accurately assess and may result in a gasless abdomen.

B. CT

Computed tomography diagnosis of small bowel obstruction is based on identifying dilated (2.5 cm or greater diameter) loops of small bowel and then recognizing a point of transition distal to which the small bowel and colon are collapsed (Figs. 3, 4, and 6). In 5% to 10% of cases, a closed loop of obstruction will be present in which the small bowel is occluded at two contiguous or adjacent locations. Adhesions are the most common cause of a closed loop of obstruction, but hernias, both internal (Fig. 7) and external, may also cause a closed loop of obstruction. Strangulated small bowel obstruction (ischemia or infarction) is almost always caused by a closed loop of obstruction. Findings that suggest ischemia are decreased mural enhancement, thickening of the bowel wall, and haziness and stranding in the contiguous mesentery and fat (Fig. 8). Mural pneumatosis and mesenteric hemorrhage are other signs of strangulation and ischemia. A "target sign," produced by submucosal edema and mucosal hyperemia, generally seen during the early phase of contrast injection,

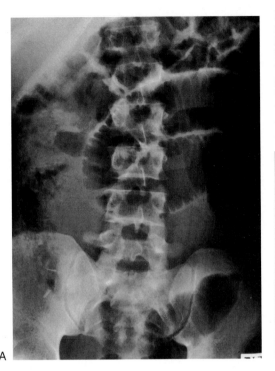

FIG. 5. Partial small bowel obstruction on plain radiography. This study shows a partial small bowel obstruction or an early complete small bowel obstruction. There is marked dilatation of the small bowel (**A** and **B**) with multiple air–fluid levels seen on the decubitus view (**B**). The colon is not dilated. Plain radiographs can be useful in the diagnosis of small bowel obstruction; however, their sensitivity, specificity, and accuracy are limited.

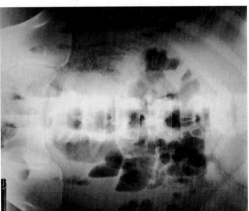

A   B

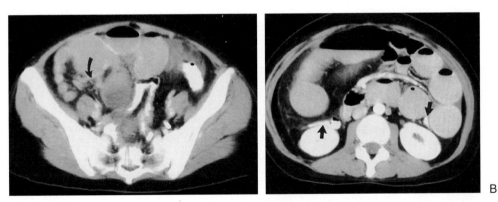

A   B

FIG. 6. Small bowel obstruction from Meckel's diverticulitis. A computed tomography scan through the pelvis **(A)** shows multiple dilated loops of small bowel. There is nondilated small bowel (*arrow*) at the point of transition. The stranding in the fat around this location is caused by the inflammation from the Meckel's diverticulum. The diverticulum itself cannot be definitively diagnosed or identified on this study. Note the nondilated colon in the right side of the pelvis in the iliac fossa. Nondilated contrast containing sigmoid is also seen near the midline. A scan at a higher level **(B)** shows multiple dilated small bowel loops with collapsed, contrast-containing ascending and descending colon (*arrows*). Contrast in the distal, nondilated bowel indicates a partial obstruction.

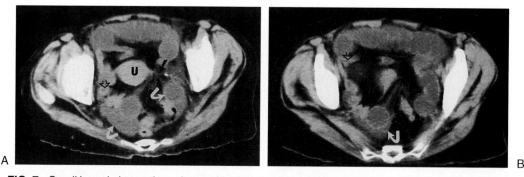

FIG. 7. Small bowel obstruction—internal hernia through left broad ligament. Computed tomography scans (**A** and **B**) through the pelvis show herniation of bowel through the left broad ligament (*arrow*). Note the dilated small bowel loops (*curved arrows*). Nondilated ileum distal to the obstruction is seen in the right pelvis (*open arrow*). Note the nondilated rectum and sigmoid (*curved arrows*). U, uterus.

may be visualized. Free extraluminal air is a sign of perforation. The actual site of perforation is usually identified. Mucosal interruption may result in mural or portal venous gas.

Incomplete obstruction may be diagnosed when there is a point of transition, with small caliber but not collapsed distal bowel (Fig. 9).

V. SENSITIVITY AND SPECIFICITY

Although a recent study by Maglinte and colleagues showed comparable accuracy for plain

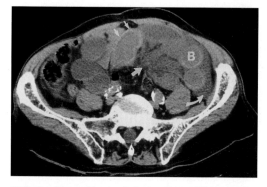

FIG. 8. Closed loop of obstruction with bowel infarction. Note dilated bowel (*B*) in left lower quadrant. High-density hematoma is evident within the leaves of the mesentery (*large arrow*). Note the high-density intramural hemorrhage within segments of the small bowel (*small arrows*). A small amount of ascitic fluid (*curved arrow*) is noted. A strangulating closed loop of obstruction with infarction of 3 feet of ileum was noted at surgery.

abdominal films and CT in diagnosing small bowel obstruction, we believe CT is probably more accurate. In the correct clinical situation, positive abdominal plain films have very high reliability in confirming the diagnosis of small bowel obstruction. Unfortunately, equivocal, false-positive and false-negative studies occur in as many as 50% of patients. When this occurs, CT is performed. CT is quite accurate in diagnosing small bowel obstruction, with reported accuracy ranging from about 70% to nearly 100%. CT can identify the cause of obstruction in 50% to 85% of patients.

VI. DIFFERENTIAL DIAGNOSIS

A. Adynamic Ileus

Adynamic ileus is best distinguished from bowel obstruction by its typically diffuse pattern of involvement in both the small bowel and colon. No point of transition is seen.

B. Acute Gastroenteritis

Acute gastroenteritis may present with crampy abdominal pain and vomiting. Radiographs show no evidence of obstruction although mild diffuse dilatation may be present.

VII. PITFALLS

When classic in their presentation, plain radiographs are useful in diagnosing small bowel

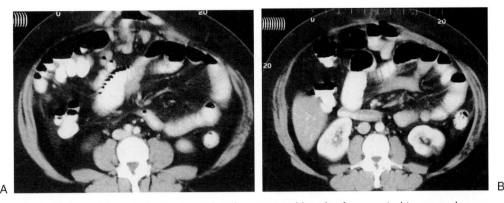

FIG. 9. Partial small bowel obstruction related to a ventral hernia. A computed tomography scan at the level of an umbilical hernia **(A)** shows bowel herniated into the subcutaneous tissue. Normal-sized bowel loops are seen exiting the region of the hernia back to the peritoneal cavity. A more cephalic scan **(B)** shows dilated loops of small bowel. Contrast is seen within the nondilated colon on both images. Findings are indicative of partial small bowel obstruction.

obstruction. Unfortunately, plain films are often nondiagnostic and can even be misleading. For this reason, CT has become more popular in the evaluation of bowel obstruction. The diagnosis is generally straightforward. It may be surprisingly difficult, however, to distinguish small bowel from colon. Although CT almost always nicely demonstrates the location of obstruction, it may be difficult to detect the cause. Presumptive diagnoses include adhesions in a postoperative patient and malignancy in a patient with cancer. These cannot always be diagnosed from the image findings alone.

VIII. SUGGESTED READINGS

Balthazar EJ, Liebeskind ME, Macari M. Intestinal ischemia in patients in whom small bowel obstruction is suspected: evaluation of accuracy, limitations, and clinical implications of CT in diagnosis. *Radiology* 1997;205:519–522.

Frager D, Medwid SW, Baer JW, Mollinelli B, Friedman M. CT of small-bowel obstruction: value in establishing the diagnosis and determining the degree and cause. *AJR Am J Roentgenol* 1994;162:37–41.

Gupta H, Dupuy DE. Advances in imaging of the acute abdomen. *Surg Clin North Am* 1997;77:1245–1263.

Maglinte DD, Reyes BL, Harmon BH, et al. Reliability and role of plain film radiography and CT in the diagnosis of small-bowel obstruction. *AJR Am J Roentgenol* 1996;167:1451–1455.

Regan F, Beall DP, Bohlman ME, Khazan R, Sufi A, Schaefer DC. Fast MR imaging and the detection of small-bowel obstruction. *AJR Am J Roentgenol* 1998;170:1465–1469.

Taourel PG, Fabre JM, Pradel JA, Seneterre EJ, Megibow AJ, Bruel JM. Value of CT in the diagnosis and management of patients with suspected acute small-bowel obstruction. *AJR Am J Roentgenol* 1995;165:1187–1192.

16

Fever and Abdominal Pain

Rule Out Abscess

Philip W. Ralls

I. CLINICAL OVERVIEW

Abdominal abscesses are most commonly encountered in patients already hospitalized after surgery, trauma, or gastrointestinal disease. More than two-thirds of abscesses are postoperative, mostly occurring because of anastomotic leaks. Perforated ulcers, biliary tract disease, and appendicitis are also common causes. Less often, an abdominal abscess presents as a primary condition. Most patients seen in the emergency department with fever and abdominal pain, however, do not have abscesses or surgical conditions.

Computed tomography (CT) is the screening examination of choice in patients with suspected abdominal abscesses because of its excellence as a survey modality and its ability to guide percutaneous aspiration and abscess drainage (Fig. 1). Sonography can be used in patients with localizing symptoms, but it is generally less sensitive than CT. Another use for sonography is to guide aspiration and drainage in patients whose abscess has been discovered by CT or other imaging modalities.

II. IMAGING STRATEGY

When an abscess is discovered, diagnostic aspiration for confirmation of the diagnosis and percutaneous abscess drainage for treatment are usually needed. CT and ultrasound, both of which can guide needle placement, are thus preferred when abscesses are sought. CT is the test of choice in all patients without localizing signs because of its excellence as a survey modality.

CT is also indicated for patients in whom an abscess is suspected but who have had negative preliminary imaging. Patients with right upper quadrant pain, right lower quadrant pain, and left lower quadrant pain can have directed imaging with ultrasound or CT to assess acute cholecystitis, appendicitis, and diverticulitis.

Other imaging tests—plain abdominal radiographs, magnetic resonance imaging, and nuclear medicine studies (gallium or labeled leukocyte studies)—are less useful. Even though their sensitivity may be adequate, they are ineffective or impractical in guiding diagnostic aspiration and percutaneous abscess drainage. Technetium 99m-labeled hexamethyl-propyleneamineoxime leukocyte or indium 111-labeled leukocyte scans may be useful if an extraabdominal abscess is suspected after a negative abdominal and pelvic CT.

III. TECHNIQUE

A. CT

Helical CT and dynamic incremental CT are both effective in seeking abdominal abscesses. An attempt should be made to opacify as much of the gastrointestinal tract as possible, including the rectum. The distal colon and rectum are usually adequately opacified when oral contrast is given 1 to 2 hours before scanning. If this lead time is not available, scanning can still be performed without giving rectal contrast. Direct opacification of the rectum is rarely necessary but can be done with air or contrast, if needed.

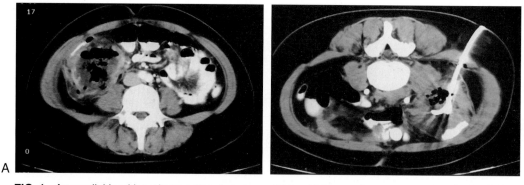

FIG. 1. Appendicitis with periappendiceal abscess. This middle-aged woman presented with abdominal pain and fever with right lower quadrant tenderness. Computed tomography revealed a gas-containing abscess in the right lower quadrant, which was presumed to represent a periappendiceal abscess **(A)**. This was subsequently drained percutaneously **(B)**.

Oral contrast is given 30 minutes before scanning and at the initiation of scanning. All scans are performed with intravenous contrast—noncontrast scans are unnecessary. We typically inject 150 mL of 60% iodinated contrast at a bolus rate of 2 to 3 cm/s with a scanning delay of 60 to 80 seconds. Scans are obtained at a 7- to 10-mm slice thickness with a table speed of 7 to 10 mm/s. For dynamic incremental CT, an injection rate of 2 mL/s is appropriate. After an 80-second delay, scans are obtained at 10-mm slice thickness and incrementation. Delayed images to opacify the renal collecting system, ureters, or bladder are occasionally useful (Fig. 2).

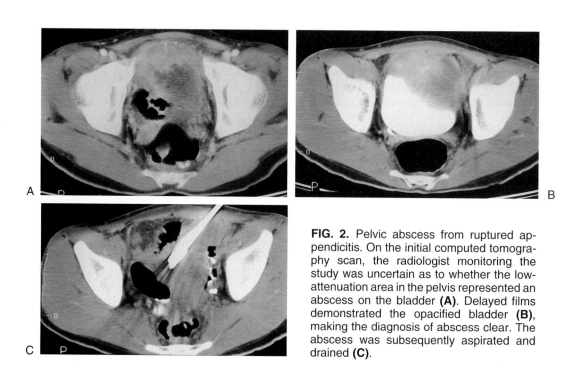

FIG. 2. Pelvic abscess from ruptured appendicitis. On the initial computed tomography scan, the radiologist monitoring the study was uncertain as to whether the low-attenuation area in the pelvis represented an abscess on the bladder **(A)**. Delayed films demonstrated the opacified bladder **(B)**, making the diagnosis of abscess clear. The abscess was subsequently aspirated and drained **(C)**.

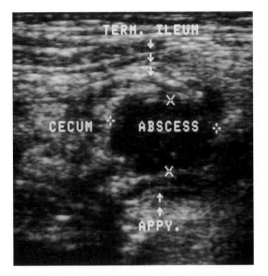

FIG. 3. Interloop abscess. The oblique transverse sonogram in the right lower abdomen shows a small interloop abscess interposed between the normal appendix and terminal ileum. Note the irregular margins and presence of debris within the predominantly hypoechoic mass. The sonographic appearance of abscesses is variable, although they are hypoechoic. Although appendicitis is a suspected cause of this abscess, the appendix was normal at surgery, as it had been on sonography. No etiology for this abscess was determined.

B. Sonography

Sonography is generally used to seek an abscess or another inflammatory condition when localizing signs are present. Because gas and bone limit it, sonography is less useful than CT as a survey modality. Careful visualization of all the areas at risk is mandatory when using sonography to seek an intraabdominal abscess. All parenchymal organs should be scanned for focal abscesses. All peritoneal spaces and interloop spaces should also be evaluated.

IV. FINDINGS

A. CT

Intraabdominal abscesses are extremely variable in appearance on CT. Abscesses most often are extraluminal fluid collections that produce a mass effect on contiguous structures (Figs. 3, 4, and 5). On occasion, abscesses may have higher attenuation. Fluid that does not displace surrounding structures is generally uninfected ascites. Gas bubbles in the lesion strongly suggest abscess, but are present in only one-third of all lesions (Figs. 1 and 6). Gas originates from gas-producing organisms or fistulous connection to the gastrointestinal tract. Needle aspiration is often required to diagnose abscess because other fluid collections (seroma, hematoma, biloma, lymphocele, pseudocyst, and others) may have nearly identical findings.

B. Sonography

Intraabdominal abscesses on sonography are typically of mixed echogenicity with a predominantly hypoechoic pattern (Figs. 7 and 8; Color Plate 7). Areas of increased echogenicity are common, usually related to gas or echogenic debris (see Fig. 3). Gas often has an associated comet-tail artifact. Abdominal abscesses may mimic solid masses (see Fig. 8).

V. SENSITIVITY AND SPECIFICITY

A. CT

The sensitivity and specificity of CT for abdominal abscess approach 100%. Percutaneous aspiration is usually necessary, however, to confirm the diagnosis.

B. Ultrasound

When unencumbered by bone, gas, or bandages, sonography has a sensitivity of more than 90% for abdominal abscess. Unfortunately, these impediments to adequate sonography are frequent, limiting the efficacy of sonography in detecting abscesses.

VI. DIFFERENTIAL DIAGNOSIS

A. Seroma

These fluid collections tend to be more homogeneous than abscesses. They are generally of water attenuation on CT and have sound trans-

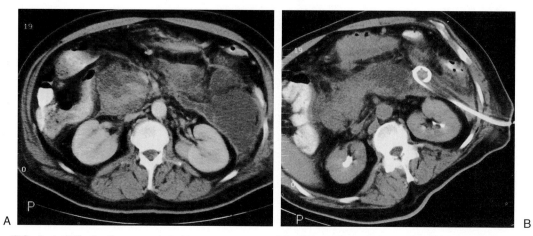

FIG. 4. Left flank abscess related to acute pancreatitis. This patient with pancreatic necrosis has a well-circumscribed left anterior perirenal space abscess **(A)**. This lesion was treated successfully with percutaneous drainage **(B)**.

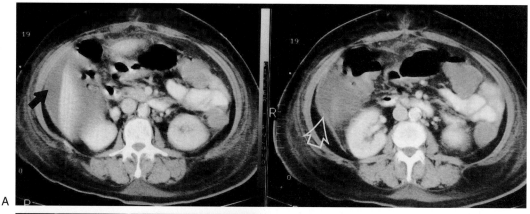

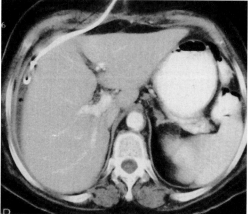

FIG. 5. Multiple abscesses after surgery. This patient developed multiple intraabdominal abscesses after repair of a perforated gastric ulcer. The computed tomography scan **(A)** performed postoperatively shows an abscess that involves the subphrenic space laterally (*arrow*) and the subhepatic and right paracolic gutter regions (*open arrow*). One week after a drain was placed in the subphrenic right paracolic gutter region, a second catheter had to be placed **(B)** to drain the persistent subphrenic abscess.

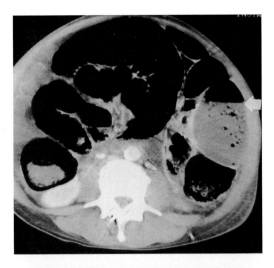

FIG. 6. Left paracolic gutter abscess. This abscess was discovered in an 57-year-old man with multiple medical problems. Note the gas suspended within the abscess and the air–fluid level (*arrow*). *Escherichia coli*, a gas-forming organism, was cultured along with several other enteric bacteria. The cause for this abscess was never determined.

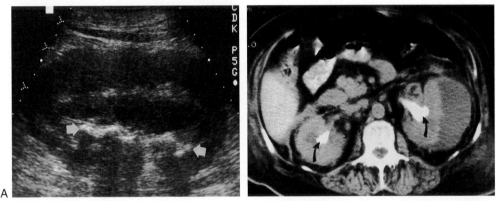

A   B

FIG. 7. Perinephric abscess. This patient presented with fever and abdominal pain. Preliminary sonography **(A)** revealed a compressed kidney with a large staghorn calculus within it (*between the arrows*). Note the subcapsular abscess that displaces the margin of the kidney (*open arrows*). The decreased echogenicity collection lateral to the renal margin is the subcapsular abscess. A computed tomography scan confirms the findings **(B)**. It also shows renal calculi in both renal pelves (*curved arrows*).

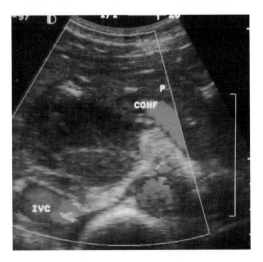

FIG. 8. Tuberculous abscess. This patient presented with fever and abdominal pain. The masslike, primarily hypoechoic abscess was detected in the juxtapancreatic region. After aspiration, this proved to be a tuberculous abscess. IVC, inferior vena cava; CONF, confluence of splenic and superior mesenteric veins; p, pancreas. (See also Color Plate 7.)

mission of sound on sonography. They tend to occur superficially in association with the surgical incision but may be deep. Aspiration may be needed in some cases to exclude an abscess.

B. Lymphocele

Lymphoceles are usually cystic or nearly cystic masses that occur in locations where surgery has disrupted normal lymphatic channels. By far the most common location is in the pelvis, medial to the iliac vessels (Fig. 9 and Color Plate 8).

C. Ascites

Ascites generally conforms to the shape of adjacent organs, without displacing them. This is true even of ascites adjacent to the readily compressible mesenteric bowel. Loculated ascites may cause a mass effect but generally has

less debris and is more homogeneous than an abscess. Septations are sometimes found in ascitic fluid with sonography.

D. Hematoma

A hematoma is generally higher in attenuation on CT than an abscess or ascites. Its distribution is peritoneal, similar to ascites, although it may cause mass effect on contiguous organs. A laminated appearance on CT suggests recurrent episodes of hemorrhage. Sonographically, hematomas are variable in appearance. Often, they have a whorled, complex mixed echogenic pattern. Acute unclotted blood or breakdown of hematoma may have an anechoic appearance. Failure to aspirate anything from an apparent fluid collection suggests hematoma. Such hematomas may be unaspiratable gel caused by a fibrin mesh.

VII. PITFALLS

Atonic fluid-filled bowel loops may simulate abscess sonographically. Bowel loops usually are identified by peristalsis on real-time images. In addition, normal bowel is compressible. On CT, unopacified loops with contents that simulate abscess (especially fecal material within the colon) can be problematic. Gas-containing abscesses can sometimes be difficult to differentiate from adjacent bowel. Delayed scans or administration of oral or rectal contrast often solves these problems.

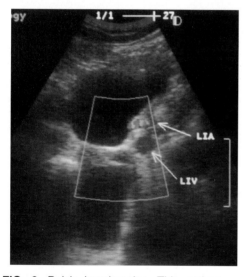

FIG. 9. Pelvic lymphoceles. This patient presented 3 weeks after pelvic surgery with a low-grade fever and pelvic pain. This fluid collection is just medial to the iliac vessels. This is the typical appearance and location for a lymphocele, although the lesion was aspirated to exclude the possibility of abscess. Another lymphocele is seen deep to the lesion contiguous with the iliac vessel. LIV, left iliac vein; LIA, left iliac artery. (See also Color Plate 8.)

VIII. SELECTED READINGS

Gazelle GS, Mueller PR. Abdominal abscess. Imaging and intervention. *Radiol Clin North Am* 1994;32:913–932.

Gupta H, Dupuy DE. Advances in imaging of the acute abdomen. *Surg Clin North Am* 1997;77:1245–1263.

Lambiase RE, Deyoe L, Cronan JJ, Dorfman GS. Percutaneous drainage of 335 consecutive abscesses: results of primary drainage with 1-year follow-up. *Radiology* 1992; 184:167–179.

Morton AM. Intraperitoneal spread of infection. In: *Dynamic radiology of the abdomen: normal and pathologic features*, 4th ed. New York: Springer-Verlag 1994:55–115.

Taourel P, Pradel J, Fabre JM, Cover S, Seneterre E, Bruel JM. Role of CT in the acute nontraumatic abdomen. *Semin Ultrasound CT MR* 1995;16:151–164.

17

Hypotension and Abdominal Pain

Rule Out Ruptured Abdominal Aortic Aneurysm

Philip W. Ralls

I. CLINICAL OVERVIEW

Rupture of an abdominal aortic aneurysm is a true catastrophe that carries a nearly 100% mortality rate if surgery is not performed urgently. Ruptured abdominal aortic aneurysm is the 15th leading cause of death of men in the United States. Its prevalence is increasing in both men and women. At least 50% of patients with ruptured abdominal aortic aneurysm die before reaching the hospital. Poor prognostic features include advanced age (over age 80), female gender, persistent hypotension, hematocrit less than 25, and transfusion requirements of more than 15 units. Preoperative cardiac arrest is associated with a survival of less than 24 hours. Obviously, successful outcome depends on accurate and early diagnosis, expeditious preoperative management, and skillful surgery.

The classic symptom triad of ruptured abdominal aortic aneurysm is abdominal or back pain, a tender abdominal mass, and hypotension. Fewer than 50% of patients, however, have the classic triad. Pain is the most frequent symptom. Rupture into the inferior vena cava with an aortocava fistula (Fig. 1 and Color Plate 9) can lead to cardiac failure, edema, and an abdominal bruit. A fistula to the gastrointestinal tract can lead to gastrointestinal hemorrhage (Fig. 2). Although most aneurysms are arteriosclerotic in etiology, mycotic aneurysms and pseudoaneurysms are sometimes encountered (Fig. 3 and Color Plate 10).

The goal of imaging is to quickly diagnose the *presence of an aneurysm*. Demonstrating signs of rupture is desirable, but only if it does not prolong the examination. Sonography is an effective and quick way to diagnose an abdominal aortic aneurysm. In more stable patients, computed tomography (CT) has been advocated as a means of evaluating these patients.

Many surgeons believe that if imaging is not immediately available, the patient should be taken to surgery, rather than risk the additional mortality associated with delay. Delayed diagnosis is correlated with increased operative mortality. Some surgeons believe it is much riskier to delay surgery than to miss a ruptured abdominal aortic aneurysm, even though operative mortality in studies reported since 1980 is still 40% to 70%.

Prophylactic surgery for treatment of a known aneurysm is a very different clinical circumstance than emergency surgery to treat a ruptured abdominal aortic aneurysm. Abdominal aortic aneurysms are generally defined as any region of abdominal aortic dilatation that exceeds a diameter of 3 cm. It is estimated that 5% of those over the age of 60 have an aneurysm by this criterion. Although aneurysms 4 cm or smaller may rupture (Fig. 4), most surgeons believe that an aneurysm of 5 cm or larger should be repaired when discovered.

II. IMAGING STRATEGY

Immediate sonography, within 5 minutes of the time the patient arrives in the emergency

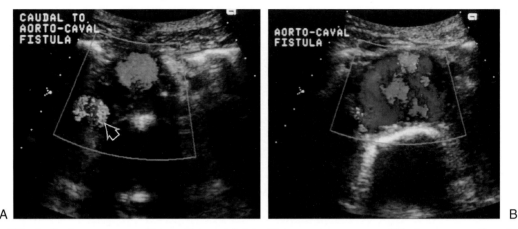

A   B

FIG. 1. Aortic aneurysm with a portocaval fistula. Transverse sonogram **(A)** shows a small aortic aneurysm with a perianeurysmal hematoma. Note that the inferior vena cava (*open arrow*) is only slightly dilated in this image obtained caudal to the site of the fistula. A sonogram near the site of the aortocaval fistula **(B)** shows marked dilatation of the inferior vena cava with turbulent flow. This patient presented with mild congestive heart failure related to the arteriovenous shunting. The exact site of the aortocaval fistula could not be demonstrated sonographically. (See also Color Plate 9.)

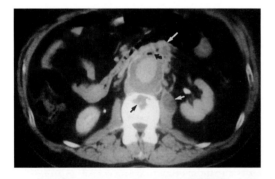

FIG. 2. Primary aortoduodenal fistula. Note the large abdominal aortic aneurysm eroding anteriorly into the duodenum. Ectopic gas (*curved black arrow*) and focal mural thickening of the posterior wall of the transverse duodenum (*long white arrow*) are evident. Also note the adjacent left psoas abscess (*short white arrow*) and lytic area in the vertebral body from posterior erosion by the aneurysm (*black arrow*). (Used with permission from Vincent McCormick, MD, San Francisco, CA.)

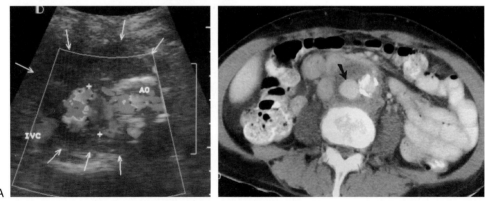

A   B

FIG. 3. Ruptured mycotic abdominal aortic aneurysm. This 56-year-old user of intravenous drugs presented with a sudden onset of lower abdominal back pain and hypotension. Color flow sonography **(A)** revealed a calcified aorta with a mycotic abdominal aortic aneurysm between the inferior vena cava (*IVC*) and aorta (*AO*). (See Color Plate 10.) A contrast-enhanced computed tomography scan **(B)** revealed the aneurysm (*arrow*) with partially surrounding clot. This patient was treated with antibiotics and surgery and survived.

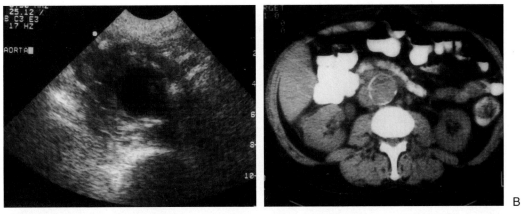

A   B

FIG. 4. Small ruptured abdominal aortic aneurysm. A 72-year-old patient with cancer presented with acute onset of abdominal pain and hypotension. A transverse sonogram **(A)** revealed a small abdominal aortic aneurysm with a periaortic abnormality indicative of hematoma. The sonographic diagnosis was ruptured abdominal aortic aneurysm. Because of clinical uncertainty, a computed tomography scan **(B)** was ordered, which again showed a small aneurysm with a perianeurysmal hematoma. The patient was taken to surgery, but died in the operating room from exsanguination. Although most ruptures occur in larger aneurysms, small aneurysms such as this one (3 cm) may also rupture with catastrophic results.

department, is optimal in patients with suspected ruptured abdominal aneurysm. The examination should not last more than 2 minutes. Remember that the focus of the examination is detection of the aneurysm, not detection of evidence of rupture. Once an aneurysm has been detected sonographically, the patient is taken to the operating room for emergency surgery. Sonography for suspected ruptured abdominal aneurysm is perhaps the most emergent imaging examination that radiologists perform. I tell our residents that if they are asked to evaluate a patient with a suspected ruptured abdominal aneurysm while they are doing an angiogram, they should immediately stop doing the angiogram to perform the ultrasound.

The delay required for other studies—angiography, dynamic CT, or magnetic resonance imaging—is generally not warranted. It is conceivable that rapid, immediately available noncontrast helical CT might be an appropriate means to evaluate patients with suspected ruptured abdominal aneurysm. This approach has not yet been evaluated.

III. TECHNIQUE

A. Ultrasound

The most important factor to remember is that sonography must be done quickly. Scanning should take no more than 2 minutes. Scanning is best performed with a large footprint curved linear transducer. Low-frequency scanning, using 3.5 MHz or lower frequency transducers, facilitates penetration. Start with the patient in the supine position. The abdominal aorta is localized using mild compression technique. Aneurysmal dilatation is sought. If there is too much gas to allow visualization in the supine position, the patient should be turned into a right lateral decubitus position— scans should be performed through the left flank. This allows visualization of the aorta along its coronal plane. The decubitus position minimizes interference from gas.

Color Doppler often facilitates the study, adds information, and does not add time to the examination.

Once an aneurysm has been detected, the ex-

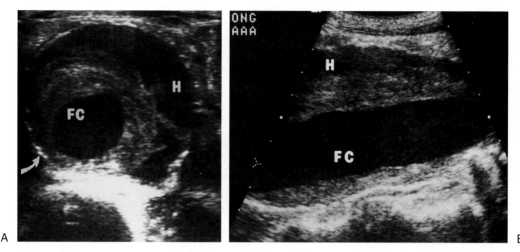

A   B

FIG. 5. Ruptured abdominal aortic aneurysm. The transverse **(A)** and longitudinal **(B)** sonograms show evidence of a ruptured abdominal aortic aneurysm. There is a large fresh hypoechoic hematoma around the aorta (*H*), partially bound by the expanded calcified aortic wall (*arrow*). A rind of clot surrounds the flow channel (*FC*). This patient was taken immediately to the operating room and survived.

amination is finished. The patient should be taken to the operating room immediately.

B. CT

A noncontrast helical CT using 10-mm collimation and 10- or 15-mm table speed should be sufficient to detect an abdominal aortic aneurysm. If time allows, intravenous contrast injection is helpful. Once again, detecting evidence of rupture is not critical, although CT is better than sonography in delineating periaortic abnormality.

IV. RADIOGRAPHIC FINDINGS

A. Ultrasound

Sonography is effective in detecting abdominal aortic aneurysm. An echogenic, calcified rim is often visible, as is a central rind of clot. Color Doppler is a helpful tool that adds no time to the examination. It detects the native aortic flow channel and delineates altered hemodynamics. An anechoic to hypoechoic region of fresh hemorrhage around the aorta may be present (Fig. 5). Crescentic clot may be seen in this hypoechoic area (Fig. 6). Regions of echogenic clot

may be seen in or near the aorta. On occasion, evidence of an aortovenous fistula may be demonstrated (see Fig. 1).

B. CT

In hemodynamically stable patients, CT can be used to demonstrate both impending and

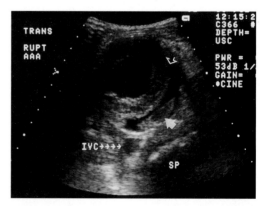

FIG. 6. Ruptured abdominal aneurysm. Transverse sonogram shows a typical "contained" rupture. Acute hemorrhage is seen outside the aortic lumen, constrained only by tissue planes and contiguous thrombus (*open arrow*). A crescentic thrombus is seen within this hematoma (*arrow*), a finding analogous to the crescent sign of rupture seen on computed tomography scans.

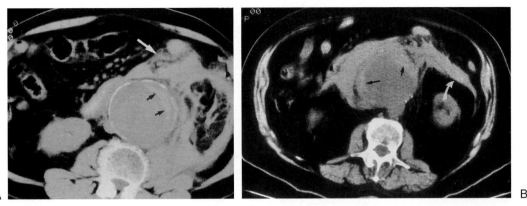

FIG. 7. Crescent sign in aortic aneurysm rupture in two patients. **A:** Note crescentic high-attenuating blood in the left anterolateral aspect of the aortic aneurysm (*black arrows*). In another patient **(B)**, note crescent sign (*black arrows*) and a large amount of hemorrhage in the anterior perineal space (*curved arrow*). (Used with permission from Leon Love, MD, Glencoe, IL.)

frank rupture of an abdominal aneurysm. One interesting CT sign of impending rupture is the so-called crescent sign, which consists of a crescentic area of high attenuation within the aortic wall (Fig. 7). The crescent sign is thought to represent acute intramural hemorrhage or hemorrhage into the mural thrombus. CT findings of rupture include extraluminal retroperitoneal blood (Fig. 8) and focal interruption of the aortic

wall. Occasionally, acute extravasation is detected (Fig. 9).

V. SENSITIVITY AND SPECIFICITY

A. Ultrasound

In Schuman's study of patients evaluated sonographically in an emergent fashion, sonogra-

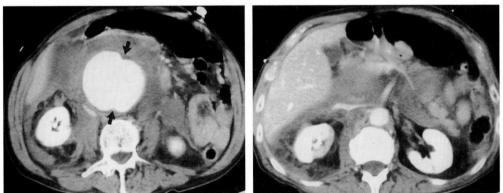

FIG. 8. Ruptured abdominal aneurysm. This patient underwent computed tomography (CT) scanning for "abdominal pain." Despite the fact that the patient was hypotensive, there was no clinical suspicion of ruptured abdominal aortic aneurysm. The CT scan **(A)** shows a rupture of this large aneurysm into the retroperitoneum. Note the dimpling (*arrow*) that likely represents the area of rupture. This hematoma extends into the retroperitoneum bilaterally and to a lesser extent into the perineal space. There is little or no hemoperitoneum. A scan higher up **(B)** reveals peripancreatic and right-sided right peritoneal hemorrhage. This patient died several weeks later because of multiple postoperative complications.

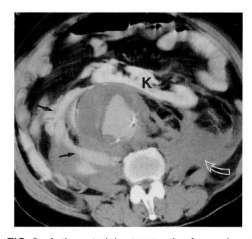

FIG. 9. Active arterial extravasation from a large abdominal aortic aneurysm. Note the extensive mural thrombus (*T*) within the aneurysm. Black arrows indicate the pathway of leakage of contrast from the lumen into the anterior perirenal space. Note the large fluid collection of high attenuation in the anterior perirenal space consistent with active arterial extravasation (*white arrow*). (Used with permission from Andrew P. Nava, MD, Salinas, CA.)

phy identified 31 of 32 abdominal aneurysms (97% sensitivity). The ultrasound examination was limited to 2 minutes in this study.

B. CT

Although data from a CT series as large as Schuman's for sonography does not exist for CT, the sensitivity of CT for detection of aneurysm should likewise be nearly 100%. CT is better in assessing periaortic abnormality and direct signs of rupture than is sonography.

VI. DIFFERENTIAL DIAGNOSIS

A. Acute Myocardial Infarction

This lacks abdominal imaging abnormalities—specifically no aneurysm is likely to be present. Obviously, the coincidental presence of an aneurysm might lead to difficulties.

Electrocardiographic abnormalities can be crucial, of course, in the differential diagnosis. Laboratory diagnosis, although delayed, is usually definitive.

B. Ureteral Stone

An aneurysm is likely to be absent. Sonography can sometimes identify a ureteral stone. More commonly, nonspecific secondary signs such as pyelocaliectasis and dilated ureters may be identified.

C. Pancreatitis

An aneurysm is likely to be absent. The pancreas is generally abnormal. Abnormalities include parenchymal heterogeneity, peripancreatic inflammation, pancreatic enlargement, or decreased pancreatic echogenicity.

D. Peptic Ulcer Disease/Perforated Ulcer

An aneurysm is likely to be absent. Sonographic findings are often sparse in this situation. Free air can sometimes be detected sonographically. An abdominal series is useful to detect free air. Water-soluble upper gastrointestinal studies are also useful to delineate the leak or abnormality associated with the ulcer.

VII. PITFALLS

There are few conditions that mimic the sonographic or CT appearance of a ruptured abdominal aortic aneurysm. The major pitfall in imaging for ruptured abdominal aortic aneurysm is detecting an aneurysm as an incidental finding in a patient who does not have rupture. The clinical condition of the patient is usually sufficient to prevent confusion. Contrast-enhanced CT is the best test to further evaluate stable patients who require additional imaging before surgery.

VIII. SUGGESTED READINGS

Adam DJ, Bradbury AW, Stuart WP, et al. The value of computed tomography in the assessment of suspected ruptured abdominal aortic aneurysm. *J Vasc Surg* 1998;27: 431–437.

Arita T, Matsunaga N, Takano K, et al. Abdominal aortic aneurysm: rupture associated with the high-attenuating crescent sign. *Radiology* 1997;204:765–768.

Johansen K, Kohler TR, Nicholls SC, Zierler RE, Clowes AW, Kazmers A. Ruptured abdominal aortic aneurysm: the Harborview experience. *J Vasc Surg* 1991;13:240–245.

Perler BA. Ruptured abdominal aortic aneurysm. In: Cameron JL, ed. *Current surgical therapy*, 5th ed. St. Louis: Mosby, 1995:621–625.

Shuman WP, Hastrup W Jr, Kohler TR, et al. Suspected leaking abdominal aortic aneurysm: use of sonography in the emergency room. *Radiology* 1988;168:117–119.

18

Acute Flank Pain

Rule Out Ureteral Calculus

R. Brooke Jeffrey, Jr.

I. CLINICAL OVERVIEW

Renal colic is a common cause of severe acute abdominal pain in clinical practice. Most patients demonstrate classic signs and symptoms that include acute flank pain radiating to the groin, nausea, and vomiting with laboratory evidence of hematuria. In the past, intravenous urography (IVU) and sonography were the primary imaging techniques used to evaluate patients with suspected renal colic. Most recently, however, noncontrast helical computed tomography (CT) has virtually replaced these two techniques as the primary method to diagnose renal or ureteral calculi. Helical CT is a much more rapid examination often requiring only 10 to 15 minutes. It involves no intravenous contrast and is more accurate than an IVU in detecting small stones. One other major benefit is the fact that noncontrast CT may be valuable in suggesting an alternative diagnosis such as appendicitis or diverticulitis when no evidence of a ureteral calculus is found.

The most important clinical questions to be answered in a patient with possible renal colic are:

1. Does the patient have a stone in the ureter?
2. If so, what is the size and location of the stone?

Eighty percent of patients with stones less than 5 mm in size will pass them spontaneously without surgical or cystoscopic intervention. Thus, in the absence of fever and suspected pyonephrosis, most patients will be treated expect- antly with analgesics and intravenous fluids. Surgery or lithotripsy is reserved for the small number of patients with larger stones that will not pass spontaneously.

II. IMAGING STRATEGY

Noncontrast helical CT is the imaging method of choice to evaluate patients with renal colic and suspected ureteral calculi. Sonography may be used in pregnant or pediatric patients to avoid ionizing radiation. In a high percentage of patients, the diagnosis of ureteral calculi can be confirmed or excluded on the basis of noncontrast CT. In a small percentage of patients, it may not be possible to differentiate a pelvic phlebolith from ureteral calculus. In this small subset of patients, intravenous contrast should be used. Intravenous injection of 50 mL of 60% contrast can be used to determine whether the calcification is located within or adjacent to the ureter. Intravenous contrast may also be extremely valuable when there is no evidence of a calculus and clinical evidence of possible pyelonephritis or renal vein thrombosis is present. In both instances there may be unilateral nephromegaly with soft tissue stranding infiltration in the perirenal fat.

Sonography is frequently used as the initial screening study for patients with fever and flank pain and suspected pyonephrosis. Typically, there is significant dilatation of the collecting system. Sonography may also then be used to guide access for percutaneous nephrostomy in cases of suspected pyonephrosis.

III. TECHNIQUE

Noncontrast helical CT scans are obtained from the T-12 vertebrae (on the top of the kidneys) and to the pubic symphysis. No oral or intravenous contrast is used. A 40-second helical acquisition is obtained using a 5-mm collimation with a pitch of 1.6. Following a brief period of deep respiratory inspiration, the patient is asked to perform a breath-held acquisition as long as possible. By starting at the kidneys and moving caudally, there is less respiratory motion moving further away from the diaphragm. Thus, the patient can perform quiet breathing after the initial breath-hold without significantly introducing motion or misregistration artifacts. After the helical acquisition, the data set is then reconstructed every 5 mm. In selected patients, it may be useful to perform either coronal or curved planar reformations. These views may occasionally help in differentiating a phlebolith from a ureteral calculus.

IV. FINDINGS

The primary findings in patients with renal colic or noncontrast CT include calcification within the renal collecting system or the ureter, nephromegaly, stranding of the perinephric fat due to forniceal rupture, and hydronephrosis or hydroureter (Figs. 1, 2, and 3). An important secondary finding that helps to differentiate a ureteral calculus from a stone is the presence of a rim of soft tissue (''tissue rim sign'') around a ureteral calculus caused by edema and local inflammation caused by the stone. The tissue rim sign is present in approximately 77% of ureteral calculi but is seen in only 8% of pelvic phleboliths.

V. SENSITIVITY AND SPECIFICITY

Smith, Rosenfield, and Choc, et al. recently reported a clinical series of noncontrast helical CT in 210 patients. The sensitivity of the CT findings was 97% with a specificity of 96%. In a subsequent article by Smith, Verga, and Dalrymple, et al. sensitivity and specificity were calculated for secondary signs of acute renal colic. Ureteral dilatation had a sensitivity of 90%, and perinephric stranding had a sensitivity of 82%. A dilated collecting system had an 83% sensitivity, whereas unilateral nephromegaly had the lowest sensitivity at 71%. A combination of several of these findings yielded very high positive predictive value. If both positive unilateral ureteral dilatation and unilateral perinephric stranding were present, the positive predictive value was 97%.

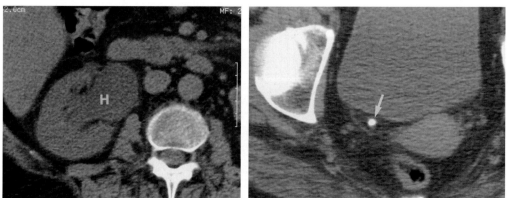

FIG. 1. Obstructing distal ureteral stone. In **(A)** note marked hydronephrosis (*H*) of the right kidney. In **(B)** note the obstructing stone in the distal right ureteropelvic junction (*arrow*).

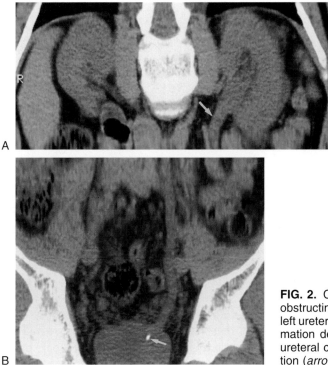

A

B

FIG. 2. Coronal reformation demonstrating obstructing distal calculus. In **(A)** note dilated left ureter (*arrow*). In **(B)** curved planar reformation demonstrates obstructing left distal ureteral calculus at the ureterovesical junction (*arrow*).

VI. DIFFERENTIAL DIAGNOSIS

A wide range of acute abdominal conditions can clinically mimic renal colic. Many of these abnormalities may be diagnosed with noncontrast helical CT during the same examination. The differential diagnosis includes diverticulitis, appendicitis (Fig. 4), ruptured aortic aneurysm (Fig. 5), and pelvic and ovarian masses (Fig. 6).

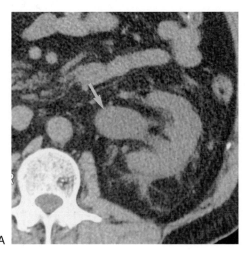

A

FIG. 3. Obstructing distal ureteral calculus with hyponephrosis and perinephric stranding. In **(A)** note the dilatation of the renal pelvis (*arrow*). *Figure continues*

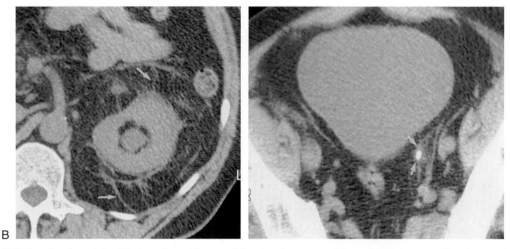

B

C

FIG. 3. *Continued.* In **(B)** there is evidence of forniceal rupture with perinephric stranding (*arrows*). In **(C)** note the distal obstructing left ureteral calculus with the tissue rim sign (*arrows*).

VII. PITFALLS

A potential pitfall with helical CT for diagnosis of renal ureteral calculi is misinterpreting a phlebolith for a ureteral calculus. The tissue rim sign is helpful in this regard because there is often soft tissue infiltration and edema around the stone impacted within the distal ureter (Fig. 7). Phleboliths do not demonstrate the tissue rim sign in a high percentage of cases (only about 8%). In problematic patients, intravenous contrast injection is required to determine the relationship of the calcification to the ureter. Another potential limitation of helical CT for renal

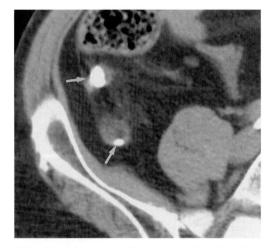

FIG. 4. Acute appendicitis clinically mimicking renal colic. Note the calcified appendicoliths (*arrows*) and adjacent periappendiceal edema within the mesoappendix indicating acute appendicitis.

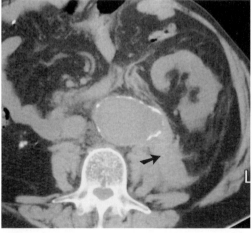

FIG. 5. Ruptured aortic aneurysm mimicking renal colic. Note high attenuation hematoma in the psoas compartment and posterior perineal space (*arrow*) from lateral rupture of calcified abdominal aortic aneurysm.

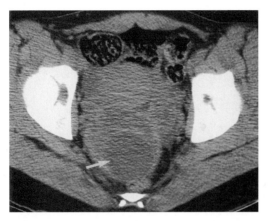

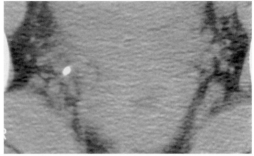

FIG. 6. Tubo-ovarian abscess mimicking renal colic. Note cystic mass in the cul-de-sac with poor definition of the posterior wall of the ureteris (*arrow*, abscess).

FIG. 8. Helical computed tomography scan indeterminate for distal right ureteral calculus. A calcification is noted adjacent to the bladder in the region of the distal right ureter. However, because of surrounding adnexal structures, it was not possible to identify the expected course of the ureter. Intravenous contrast injection demonstrated that the stone was indeed within the ureter.

colic is that it does not provide any physiologic information about the degree of ureteral obstruction (Fig. 8). However, in a vast majority of patients, the critical features for initial manage-

ment are the size and location of the stone. Intravenous contrast should be used routinely to evaluate for pyelonephritis and renal masses. It is important to obtain delayed images (5 to 10 minutes) after contrast injection to optimally detect renal masses.

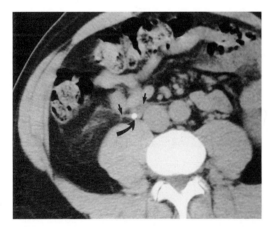

FIG. 7. Tissue rim sign of ureteral calculus. Note calculus in right midureter (*curved arrow*). There is thickening of the wall of the ureter with periureteral soft tissue stranding (*arrows*).

VIII. SUGGESTED READINGS

Katz DS, Lane MJ, Sommer FG. Unenhanced helical CT of ureteral stones: incidence of associated urinary tract findings. *AJR Am J Radiol* 1996;166:1319–1322.

Smith RC, Rosenfield AT, Choc KA, et al. Acute flank pain: comparison of non-contrast-enhanced CT and intravenous urography. *Radiology* 1995;194:789–794.

Smith RC, Verga M, Dalrymple N, McCarthy S, Rosenfield AT. Acute ureteral obstruction: value of secondary signs on helical unenhanced CT. *AJR Am J Radiol* 1996;167:1109–1113.

Smith RC, Verga M, McCarthy S, Rosenfield AT. Diagnosis of acute flank pain: value of unenhanced helical CT. *AJR Am J Radiol* 1996;166:97–101.

Sommer FG, Jeffrey RB Jr, Rubin GD, et al. Detection of ureteral calculi in patients with suspected renal colic: value of reformatted noncontrast helical CT. *AJR Am J Radiol* 1995;165:509–513.

19

Acute Pelvic Pain and Positive β-Human Chorionic Gonadotropin

Rule Out Ectopic Pregnancy

R. Brooke Jeffrey, Jr.

I. CLINICAL OVERVIEW

Ectopic pregnancy is increasing in incidence due to the continued epidemic of pelvic inflammatory disease and the growing number of patients undergoing in vitro fertilization for infertility. Although the mortality rate related to ectopic pregnancy is declining, it nevertheless represents 15% of all maternal deaths. All women of childbearing age should be considered at risk for ectopic pregnancy. This fact should always be kept in mind whenever pelvic sonography is performed for any acute symptoms. More specific risk factors for an ectopic pregnancy include a prior ectopic pregnancy, pelvic inflammatory disease, prior tubal reconstructive surgery, intrauterine contraceptive devices, and increased maternal age and parity. The use of antimetabolites (e.g., methotrexate) represents an important new advance in the pharmacologic treatment for unruptured tubal pregnancies and has substantially decreased the number of operative procedures for this condition. Although 95% of all ectopic pregnancies are located within the fallopian tubes, it is important to diagnose cornual (interstitial) and intraabdominal ectopic pregnancies because of their significantly higher morbidity.

II. IMAGING STRATEGY

Sonography remains the imaging method of choice in all patients with suspected ectopic pregnancy. Transabdominal and endovaginal scanning should be performed routinely. Endovaginal sonography is clearly superior, however, in demonstrating subtle features within the endometrial cavity and adnexa. Color flow imaging is an important adjunct to gray-scale sonography and may be of value in identifying a high-velocity, low-resistance flow pattern (peritrophoblastic flow) associated with an ectopic pregnancy.

III. SONOGRAPHIC TECHNIQUE

Imaging of the upper abdomen including the right paracolic gutter and hepatorenal fossa should be performed routinely with standard abdominal (3.5- to 5-MHz) transducers. It is important to survey the upper abdomen to evaluate for hemoperitoneum extending from the pelvis into the upper peritoneal spaces. In a patient with a full bladder, preliminary scans may be obtained in longitudinal transverse planes of the uterus and adnexa. In the absence of a full urinary bladder, endovaginal scanning should be immediately performed rather than waiting for the bladder to fill from intravenous fluids. Endovaginal scanning is generally performed using a 5- to 7-MHz transducer. Images are obtained of the endometrial cavity, the ovaries, and adnexal regions. Color Doppler sonography with spectral Doppler tracings is useful to evaluate adnexal masses. The demonstration of extrauterine high-velocity and low-resistance flow around an

183

echogenic adnexal ring is typical of peritrophoblastic flow associated with an ectopic gestation.

IV. FINDINGS

The most important imaging observation to make in a patient with a suspected ectopic pregnancy is to "rule-in" an intrauterine pregnancy (IUP) (Figs. 1–5). Identification of an IUP dramatically diminishes the potential chance of an ectopic pregnancy. A coexistent IUP with an ectopic pregnancy is estimated to occur in 1 of 7,000 pregnancies. The most highly reliable finding of an IUP on endovaginal sonography is identification of a live embryo with a beating heart. The identification of a yolk sac is also a highly reliable finding of an IUP. Prior to 6 or 7 weeks of gestation two more subtle findings indicate an IUP and require some experience to interpret. These include the intradecidual sign and double decidual sign of the IUP.

The intradecidual sign (see Fig. 3) refers to an echogenic sac within the decidua located adjacent to and abutting the endometrial canal. It must be distinguished from a decidual cyst that may be associated with ectopic pregnancy. Decidual cysts typically are not bordered by an echogenic ring and are located deep within the decidua not adjacent to the endometrial canal (Fig. 6). The double decidual sign refers to an inner echogenic ring formed by the decidua capsularis and chorion laeve that is surrounded by a

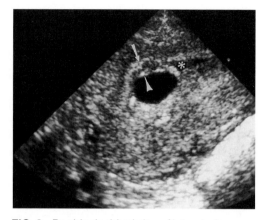

FIG. 2. Double decidual sign of intrauterine pregnancy. An endovaginal sonogram demonstrates an early intrauterine pregnancy. Note the two echogenic rings. The inner echogenic ring (*arrowhead*) represents the decidual capsularis and the outer echogenic ring (*arrow*) represents the decidual parietalis. Note the small amount of fluid within the endometrial cavity (*). (Case courtesy of Faye Laing, MD, Boston, MA.)

second echogenic ring representing the decidua parietalis. The above finding should be distinguished from the potential pitfall of a simple endometrial fluid collection (decidua cast) that is surrounded by a single layer of decidua.

When the mean sac diameter is 8 mm, a clearly visible yolk sac should be evident with

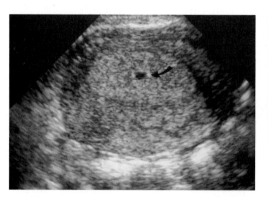

FIG. 1. Early intrauterine pregnancy before the development of a yolk sac. Note the small gestational sac bordered by an echogenic ring (*arrow*).

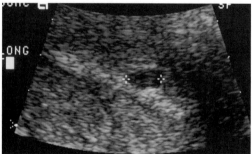

FIG. 3. Intradecidual sign of early intrauterine pregnancy. Note the gestational sac (*cursors*) embedded within the endometrium adjacent to the endometrial stripe. Fluid within the endometrial cavity would not be centrally extrinsically positioned. Therefore, this represents an early intrauterine pregnancy.

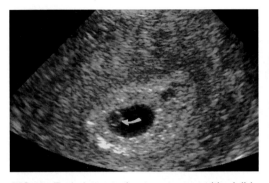

FIG. 4. Early intrauterine pregnancy with visible yolk sac. Note the yolk sac (*arrow*) within the gestational sac on this endovaginal sonogram.

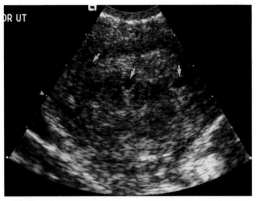

FIG. 6. Decidual cysts associated with ectopic pregnancy. Endovaginal sonogram reveals multiple decidual cysts (*arrows*). Note the multiple decidual cysts that lack contiguity with the endometrial cavity.

endovaginal sonography. By the time the mean sac diameter is 16 mm, an embryo should always be visualized. Failure to visualize a yolk sac or embryo by these landmarks generally indicates an abnormal IUP such as a blighted ovum.

Another point to remember is that unruptured tubal pregnancies may have no abnormal sonographic findings. A normal scan therefore should not be misconstrued as definitive evidence "excluding" an ectopic pregnancy. It has been estimated that up to one-third of patients with ectopic pregnancy demonstrate no adnexal pathology and no cul-de-sac fluid using endovaginal sonography.

Adnexal findings in patients with ectopic pregnancies include masses (a combination of hematosalpinx or clotted hemoperitoneum) (Fig. 7), an echogenic tubal ring representing the ectopic gestation (Fig. 8), and identification of an extrauterine embryo. Although a nonspecific finding, the presence of free intraperitoneal fluid with low-level echo suggests hemoperitoneum (Fig. 9). Clotted blood may be relatively echogenic and demonstrate masslike effect. In com-

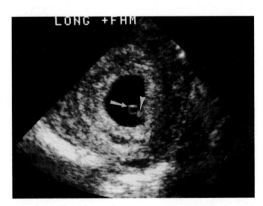

FIG. 5. Early intrauterine pregnancy with visible embryo. Endovaginal scan demonstrates the yolk sac (*arrow*) and embryo with a positive heartbeat on real-time imaging (*arrowhead*). (Case courtesy of Faye Laing, MD, Boston, MA.)

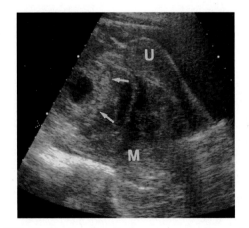

FIG. 7. Ruptured ectopic pregnancy. Transabdominal sonogram demonstrates large retrouterine complex mass (*M*) representing clotted blood in the cul-de-sac. The clotted blood displaces the uterus (*U*) anteriorly. Note echogenic ring (*arrows*) of ectopic gestation.

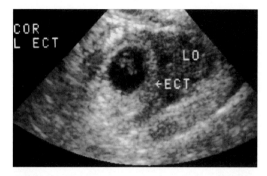

FIG. 8. Unruptured ectopic pregnancy. Note ectopic material (*ECT*) with echogenic ring adjacent to the left ovary (*LO*). An embryo is present within the ectopic gestational sac but there was no visible heartbeat.

bination with an adnexal mass, echogenic free fluid has a 97% positive predictive value for ectopic pregnancy.

V. SENSITIVITY AND SPECIFICITY

The most specific finding of ectopic pregnancy is the demonstration of an extrauterine embryo with a beating heart. This has been reported to be detected in 17% to 28% of patients

using endovaginal sonography. In patients with unruptured ectopic pregnancies, an echogenic tubal ring is a frequent finding. It has been reported in 68% of patients with unruptured tubal pregnancy. The identification of a tubal ring has nearly 100% positive predictive value for ectopic pregnancy.

VI. DIFFERENTIAL DIAGNOSIS

In the setting of a positive pregnancy test, the differential diagnosis of adnexal masses is limited. An ectopic pregnancy must be considered in the absence of an IUP. Hemoperitoneum may be caused by a ruptured corpus luteal cyst and not an ectopic pregnancy. Other echogenic pelvic masses include a dermoid cyst, ovarian torsion, hemorrhagic cyst, and clotted hemoperitoneum (Fig. 10). A pyosalpinx may contain echogenic pus that may simulate a hematosalpinx. The identification of high-velocity, lower-resistance flow (the "ring of fire") surrounding an extraovarian adnexal mass with an echogenic ring strongly suggests ectopic pregnancy (Fig. 11 and Color Plate 11). However, in the absence of specific Doppler parameters of low-resistance flow, ectopic pregnancy cannot be excluded.

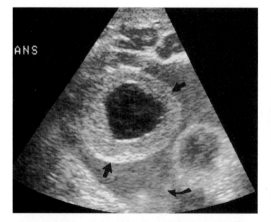

FIG. 9. Ruptured ectopic pregnancy with echogenic hemoperitoneum. Endovaginal sonogram demonstrates echogenic ring surrounding ectopic gestational sac and right adnexa (*arrows*). The ectopic material is surrounded by echogenic fluid (*curved arrow*) representing hemoperitoneum.

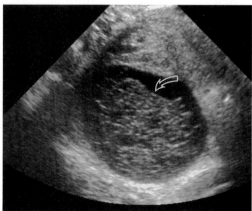

FIG. 10. Hemorrhagic functional cyst. Note echogenic clot within a right adnexal cyst. Clues to the fact that there was internal hemorrhage within the cyst include the fact that it was avascular in color Doppler and had a straight margin representing clot retraction.

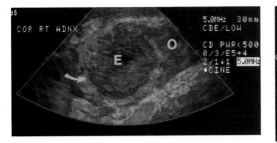

FIG. 11. Peritrophoblastic flow surrounding ectopic pregnancy. Note the echogenic ring of an ectopic pregnancy (*E*) adjacent to the right ovary. Power Doppler demonstrates peritrophoblastic flow around the ectopic gestation (*curved arrow*). (See also Color Plate 11.)

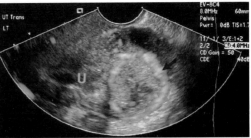

FIG. 13. Cornual (interstitial) ectopic pregnancy with peritrophoblastic flow. Endovaginal scan of the uterus demonstrates peritrophoblastic flow around the cornual ectopic gestation along the left lateral margin of the uterus (*U*). (See also Color Plate 12.)

VII. PITFALLS

Unless the findings are clear-cut, it is important not to attempt to "overdiagnose" an early intrauterine pregnancy in the absence of an embryo or a yolk sac. It requires some experience in correctly interpreting both the intradecidual and the double decidual sign. Whenever in doubt, it is prudent to cautiously err on the side of not being able to "exclude an ectopic pregnancy" and to follow the patient carefully with serial human chorionic gonadotropin tests and follow-up sonograms. Although 95% of ectopic pregnancies occur in the ampullary portion of the tube, a cornual or interstitial location occurs in approximately 2% to 5%. This is located at the junction of the endometrial cavity and the fallopian tubes. Due to its intramural location, cornual ectopic pregnancies may cause massive hemoperitoneum because of enlarged myometrial vessels that may rupture (Figs. 12 and 13; Color Plate 12). Because of the high morbidity and mortality of cornual ectopic pregnancy, early diagnosis is critically important for this rare but clinically significant variation. A cornual or interstitial pregnancy will not demonstrate a double sac sign but will often be directly connected to the intermedial cavity via the "interstitial line sign" as the eccentrically positioned intramural pregnancy abuts the endometrial cavity.

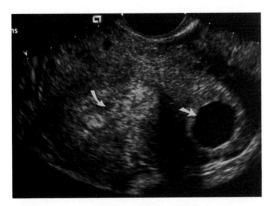

FIG. 12. Cornual (interstitial) ectopic pregnancy. Endovaginal scan demonstrates cornual ectopic gestational sac (*arrow*). Note endometrial stripe (*curved arrow*).

VIII. SUGGESTED READINGS

Ackerman TE, Levi CS, Dashefsky SM, et al. Interstitial line: sonographic finding in interstitial (cornual) ectopic pregnancy. *Radiology* 1993;189:83.

Filly RA. Ultrasound evaluation during the first trimester. In: Callen PW, ed. *Ultrasonography in obstetrics and gynecology*, 3rd ed. Philadelphia, WB Saunders, 1994:63.

Nyberg DA, Filly RA, Laing FC, et al. Ectopic pregnancy: diagnosis by sonography correlated with quantitative HCG levels. *J Ultrasound Med* 1987;6:145.

Nyberg DA, Laing FC, Filly RA, et al. Ultrasonographic differentiation of the gestational sac of early intrauterine pregnancy from the pseudogestational sac of ectopic pregnancy. *Radiology* 1983;146:755.

Pellerito JS, Taylor KJW, Quedens-Case C, et al. Ectopic pregnancy: evaluation with endovaginal colour flow imaging. *Radiology* 1992;183:407.

20

Acute Pelvic Pain

Rule Out Adnexal Torsion

R. Brooke Jeffrey, Jr.

I. CLINICAL OVERVIEW

Adnexal torsion should always be considered in the differential diagnosis of a female patient with acute pelvic pain. The pain may be severe or intermittent due to detorsion. Benign cystic masses such as hemorrhagic cysts, cystic teratomas, and the like may be associated with ovarian torsion. It is exceedingly rare, however, for ovarian carcinomas to torse. Torsion, however, may occur in the absence of a mass and involve the normal ovary and adnexa. Torsion may also occur in the setting of hyperstimulated ovaries caused by infertility drugs. Prompt surgery with detorsion or ovarian cystectomy can result in a high percentage of ovarian salvage if untwisting of the adnexa is accomplished before infarction occurs.

II. IMAGING STRATEGY

Sonography performed with both transabdominal and endovaginal probes is the technique of choice in evaluating patients with acute pelvic pain and suspected torsion. Magnetic resonance imaging or computed tomography (or both) may be used in problematic cases if there is concern for other abnormalities such as appendicitis, diverticulitis, ureteral calculi, or other acute pelvic pathology.

III. TECHNIQUE

Transabdominal sonography using a full-bladder technique as well as endovaginal scans of the uterus and adnexa should be routinely performed in patients with possible torsion. Color Doppler sonography combined with spectral Doppler waveform analysis may be of value in assessing adnexal masses and determining whether there is central venous flow, which is characteristic of acute severe torsion.

IV. FINDINGS

Ovarian torsion may or may not be associated with a pelvic mass. In general, an enlarged but otherwise identifiable ovary is noted (Fig. 1). In some patients, the main clue to torsion is an extrapelvic location of the ovary or a mass. A typical extrapelvic location is between the uterus and bladder (Figs. 2 and 3). The gray-scale and Doppler findings in torsed ovaries are variable and depend on the degree of vascular compromise and necrosis and whether there is an associated mass. In many patients, the ovary is significantly enlarged (the normal ovary measures $3 \times 2.5 \times 1.5$ cm) and contains prominent peripheral follicles (see Fig. 1). Prominent peripheral follicles are due to the increased ovarian interstitial pressure from venous outflow obstruction that leads to transudation of fluid into immature follicles. Parenchymal edema and hemorrhage may result in increased echogenicity of the enlarged ovary. Infarction and necrosis of the ovary result in discrete cystic areas within the enlarged ovary. An extrapelvic location of the torsed ovary is a frequent finding in prepubertal girls (see Fig. 3). The

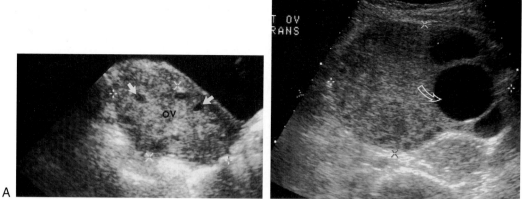

FIG. 1. Adnexal torsion in two patients. **A:** A sonogram of the right ovary in a 9-year-old girl demonstrates an enlarged echogenic ovary (*OV*) with well-visualized peripheral follicles (*arrows*). **B:** In another patient with torsion, note marked ovarian enlargement (*cursors*) and prominent peripheral follicles (*arrow*).

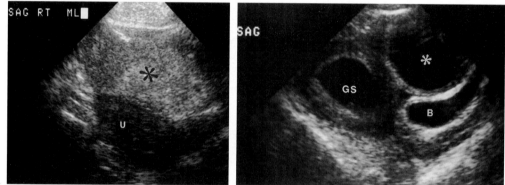

FIG. 2. Extrapelvic location of torsed ovary in two patients. **A:** Note an echogenic dermoid cyst that has undergone torsion (*) and is located anterior to the uterus (*U*). **B:** In another patient the urinary bladder (*B*) is compressed by a large cyst (*) that has undergone torsion anterior to the gravid uterus with a gestation sac (*GS*). (Case courtesy of Faye Laing, MD, Boston, MA.)

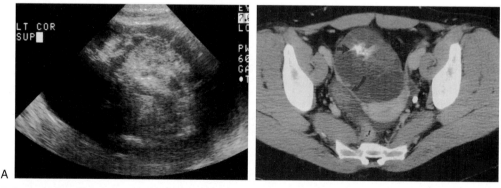

FIG. 3. Torsed ovary with dermoid cyst anterior to the uterus. **A:** Note a large echogenic mass seen anteriorly within the abdomen. **B:** A computed tomography scan demonstrates the anterior location of the mass. The mass contains internal calcifications (*arrow*) characteristic of a dermoid (*arrow*). There is stretching of the broad ligament (*curved arrow*) on the right due to the extrapelvic location of the torsed ovary.

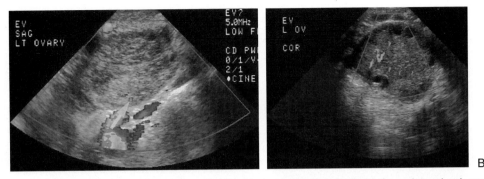

FIG. 4. Torsed ovary with preserved arterial flow in two patients. **A:** Note the enlarged echogenic left ovary with peripheral color Doppler signals still evident (*arrow*). Low-amplitude arterial waveforms were obtained from this small vessel. **B:** In another patient, the preserved arterial flow is more centrally within the torsed left ovary on this endovaginal color Doppler. No central venous flow was obtained. (See also Color Plate 13.)

torsed ovary may be located immediately anterior to the uterus.

The ovary has a dual arterial supply with one feeding branch (the ovarian artery) directly from the aorta and a second arterial feeder from the ovarian branch of the uterine artery. In a completely infarcted ovary no flow will be detected with color Doppler. In an ischemic but not infarcted ovary arterial flow (particularly within capsular branches) may still be preserved (Fig. 4 and Color Plate 13). Central venous flow is generally absent with more advanced ischemia. If the ovary detorses and the patient's symptoms subside, hyperemic flow due to reperfusion may be observed with color Doppler (Fig. 5 and Color Plate 14).

V. SENSITIVITY AND SPECIFICITY

To date, most of the clinical series documenting torsion have been relatively small and, therefore, there are few data regarding the actual sensitivity and specificity of sonography and the diagnosis of ovarian torsion.

VI. DIFFERENTIAL DIAGNOSIS

The differential diagnosis of ovarian torsion primarily includes other causes of acute pelvic pain. These are intracystic hemorrhage within either a functional cyst or an endometrioma, pel-

vic inflammatory disease, ureteral calculi, and appendicitis or other gastrointestinal disorders, such as bowel obstruction or diverticulitis.

VII. PITFALLS

Other pelvic masses such as dermoid cysts, degenerating fibroids, and tubo-ovarian abscesses may at times mimic the sonographic ap-

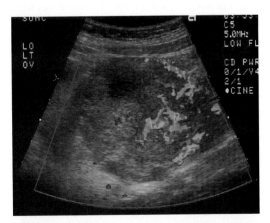

FIG. 5. Reperfusion of a torsed ovary following detorsion. This patient had severe left lower quadrant pain that suddenly subsided. A color Doppler image of the left ovary demonstrates an enlarged ovary with prominent internal flow. Over a period of several weeks, the ovary reduced in size. This likely represents detorsion with associated increased profusion. (See also Color Plate 14.)

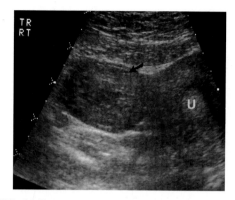

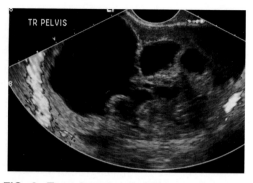

FIG. 6. Degenerating myoma mimicking ovarian torsion. Transverse scan of the right adnexa demonstrates moderately echogenic mass attached to the uterus (*U*). Surgery revealed a degenerating myoma of the broad ligament (*arrow, myoma*).

FIG. 8. Torsed ovary mimicking ovarian carcinoma. Note the complex adnexal mass on this endovaginal sonogram. Large cystic areas (*arrows*) corresponded at pathology to areas of liquefactive necrosis. A clue to the diagnosis was the fact that no flow was demonstrated within the mass with color Doppler imaging.

pearance of a torsed ovary (Fig. 6). Ovarian enlargement may also be secondary to oophoritis from pelvic inflammatory disease (Fig. 7) or polycystic ovaries. A hemorrhagic cyst has a fairly characteristic sonographic appearance as a "fishnet" pattern due to interlacing strands of fibrin. Endometriomas, depending on the acuity of internal hemorrhage, may have a variable appearance.They characteristically appear as discrete cystic masses with uniform mid- to low-level homogeneous echoes.

If detorsion occurs, increased perfusion of the

ovary may be noted depending on the timing of the color Doppler examination (see Fig. 5). The presence of central venous flow within a torsed ovary is a useful sign indicating a potentially viable torsed ovary. Surgical intervention to detorse the torsed ovary in this setting has a high degree of success. In a small group of patients with torsion, extensive liquefactive necrosis results in a complex cystic mass that may mimic the sonographic appearance of an ovarian neoplasm (Fig. 8). One clue to the diagnosis is that ovarian malignancies tend to have increased diastolic flow with low resistive indices on spectral Doppler. A torsed ovary, in contrast, typically demonstrates either no arterial flow or dampened diastolic flow with high resistive indices.

VIII. SUGGESTED READINGS

Helvie MA, Silver TM. Ovarian torsion: sonographic evaluation. *J Clin Ultrasound* 1989;17:327–332.

Kimura I, Togashi K, Kawakami S, et al. Ovarian torsion: CT and MR imaging appearances. *Radiology* 1994;190: 337–341.

Rosado WM Jr, Trambert MA, Gosink BB, et al. Adnexal torsion: diagnosis by using Doppler sonography. *AJR Am J Radiol* 1992;159:1251–1253.

Stark JE, Siegel MJ. Ovarian torsion in prepubertal girls and pubertal girls: sonographic findings. *AJR Am J Radiol* 1994;163:1479–1482.

Van Voorhis BJ, Schwaiger J, Syrop CH, et al. Early diagnosis of ovarian torsion by color Doppler sonography. *Fertil Steril* 1992;58:215–217.

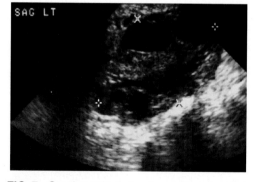

FIG. 7. Ovarian enlargement secondary to pelvic inflammatory disease. Note enlarged left ovary containing multiple fluid collections representing either abscesses or enlarged follicles. (Case courtesy of Faye Laing, MD, Boston, MA.)

Subject Index

Note: Page references to figures are italicized.
Page references to tables are followed by a *t*.

A

Abdominal abscess, 163–168
  acute pancreatitis with, *164*
  clinical overview of, 163, *164*
  differential diagnosis of, 168
  imaging findings, *164–167,* 165
  imaging pitfalls, 168
  imaging sensitivity and specificity, 165, 168
  imaging strategy, 163
  imaging technique, 163–165, *164*
  interloop, *165*
  postoperative, *166*
Abdominal aortic aneurysm
  ruptured. *See* Ruptured abdominal aortic aneurysm
  ruptured mycotic, *171*
Abdominal pain. *See* Ruptured abdominal aortic
    aneurysm
  acute. *See* Acute pancreatitis
  crampy. *See* Small bowel obstruction
Abdominal radiography
  of abdominal abscess, 163
  of small bowel obstruction, 155
    findings, 158, *159*
    sensitivity and specificity, 155, 160
    strategy, 155–156
    technique, 157
Abdominal trauma
  blunt. *See* Blunt abdominal trauma
Abscess
  abdominal. *See* Abdominal abscess
  brain, *36–38*
  epidural, *62*
  hepatic, *145*
  hypoechoic, *136*
  interloop, *165*
  mural, *126*
  paracolic gutter, *167*
  pelvic, 143, *144*
    from ruptured appendicitis, *164*
  periappendiceal, *136*
    appendicitis with, *164*
  pericholecystic
    acute cholecystitis with, 121–122, *123*

  peridiverticular, 143, *143*
  perinephric, *167*
  right upper quadrant, 131
  tuberculous, *167*
  tubo-ovarian, 137, *137*
    mimicking renal colic, 179, *180*
Acalculous cholecystitis
  acute, 119, 121–122, *121–122*
  gangrenous, *121, 122*
Acanthoamoeba, 50
Acquired immunodeficiency syndrome, 39, *44*
Actinomycosis, 79, *82*
Acute abdominal pain. *See* Acute pancreatitis
Acute acalculous cholecystitis, 119, 121–122,
    121–122
Acute appendicitis. *See* Appendicitis
Acute chest pain of noncardiac origin, 77–84
  clinical overview of, 77–78
  differential diagnosis of, 83
  imaging findings, 79, *79–83,* 83
  imaging pitfalls, 83–84
  imaging sensitivity and specificity, 83
  imaging strategy, 78–79
  imaging technique, 79
Acute cholecystitis, 119–131
  clinical overview of, 119, *120*
  differential diagnosis of, 130–131
  imaging pitfalls, 131
  imaging strategy, 119, 121–122, *121–122*
  imaging technique, 122–130, *122–130*
  with pericholecystic abscess, 121–122, *123*
  radiographic findings, 126, *126–129*
Acute disseminated encephalomyelitis (ADEM),
    46, *48*
Acute diverticulitis, 141–148
  clinical overview of, 141
  differential diagnosis of, 145–148, *146–148*
  with free air, 143, *144*
  imaging pitfalls, *146,* 148
  imaging sensitivity and specificity, 143, 145
  imaging strategy, 141–142
  imaging technique, 142
  radiographic findings, 142–143, *142–145*
Acute eosinophilic pneumonia (AEP), 85
Acute flank pain. *See* Ureteral calculi
Acute gastroenteritis, 161

postinfectious, 53
transverse, 55, *56*
viral, *55*
Myelogram
of necrotizing amebic myelitis, *50*
Myelopathy
acute. *See* Acute myelopathy
traumatic, 58, *59–60*
Myoma
degenerating
mimicking ovarian torsion, 192, *192*

N

Nasogastric tube, 105, 106
Necrotizing amebic myelitis, *50*
Necrotizing pancreatitis, 149–152, *151*
Necrotizing pneumonia, 87
Needle aspiration
of abdominal abscess, 165
Neoplastic disease, 85–86, *92*
Non-small-cell carcinoma, 92
Nonsteroidal anti-inflammatory agents, 58
Nuclear medicine studies
of abdominal abscess, 163

O

Obstructive atelectasis, *72,* 86, *90*
Occult head trauma, *9*
Osteomyelitis
tubercular vertebral, *63*
Ovarian carcinoma
adnexal torsion mimicking, 192, *192*
Ovarian enlargement
secondary to pelvic inflammatory disease, 192, *192*
Ovarian torsion. *See* Adnexal torsion

P

Pain
abdominal. *See* Ruptured abdominal aortic aneurysm
acute flank. *See* Ureteral calculi
acute pelvic. *See* Ectopic pregnancy
chest
cause of, 78
esophageal, 78
left lower quadrant. *See* Acute diverticulitis
right lower quadrant. *See* Appendicitis
right upper quadrant. *See* Acute cholecystitis
Pancoast tumor, 79, 83, *83*
Pancreatic carcinoma
mimicking acute pancreatitis, 153, *153*
Pancreatic hemorrhage, *150*

Pancreatic laceration, 116
Pancreatic necrosis, *150*
with abdominal abscess, *164*
Pancreatic pseudocysts, 152, *152*
cystic pancreatic metastases mimicking, 153, *153*
Pancreatitis, 174
acute, 130
edematous, *150,* 150–151
necrotizing, 149
Paracolic gutter abscess, *167*
Paranasal sinus infection, 34
Paraplegia, 54
Paravertebral cavity, 71, *71*
Paravertebral hematoma, 73, *75*
Parenchymal bacterial infection, 45
Parenchymal cerebritis, 34
Parenchymal disease
pulmonary, 108–109, *108–109*
Parenchymal hemorrhage, *2–3,* 5, 85, *101*
Parenchymal infarction, *99*
Parenchymal laceration, 71, *71*
Parenchymal tear, 71
Pelvic abscess, 143, *144*
from ruptured appendicitis, *164*
Pelvic inflammatory disease, 147–148, *147–148*
ovarian enlargement secondary to, 192, *192*
Pelvic lymphoceles, 168, *168*
Pelvic pain
acute. *See* Adnexal torsion; Ectopic pregnancy
Penetrating chest trauma, 65, 66
Peptic ulcer disease, 174–175
Perforated duodenal ulcer, 130–131
Perforated sigmoid diverticulitis, 143, *144*
Periappendiceal abscess, *136*
appendicitis with, *164*
Pericholecystic abscess
acute cholecystitis with, 122, *123*
Pericholecystic inflammation, *124, 126*
Pericolonic hyperemia, *145*
Pericolonic inflammation, 142, *142*
Peridiverticular abscess, 143, *143, 146*
Perinephric abscess, *167*
Perinephric stranding
ureteral calculus with, 178, *179*
Peripancreatic fluid collections, *151,* 151–152
Peritrophoblastic flow
ectopic pregnancy with, 187, *187*
Phlebolith
misinterpreted as ureteral calculus, 180
Pleural effusion, *84*
Pleural empyema, 78

3